Talking to Your Doctor

Talking to Your Doctor

A Patient's Guide to Communication in the Exam Room and Beyond

Zackary Berger

ROWMAN & LITTLEFIELD PUBLISHERS, INC.
Lanham • Boulder • New York • Toronto • Plymouth, UK

Published by Rowman & Littlefield Publishers, Inc.
A wholly owned subsidiary of The Rowman & Littlefield Publishing Group, Inc.
4501 Forbes Boulevard, Suite 200, Lanham, Maryland 20706
www.rowman.com

10 Thornbury Road, Plymouth PL6 7PP, United Kingdom

British Library Cataloguing in Publication Information Available

Library of Congress Cataloging-in-Publication Data

Berger, Zackary, 1973-
Talking to your doctor : a patient's guide to communication in the exam room and beyond / Zackary Berger.
p. cm.
Includes bibliographical references and index.
ISBN 978-1-4422-2050-8 (cloth : alk. paper) -- ISBN 978-1-4422-2051-5 (electronic)
1. Patient participation. 2. Physician and patient. 3. Communication in medicine. I. Title.
R727.42.B47 2013
610.69'6--dc23

2013014172

™ The paper used in this publication meets the minimum requirements of American National Standard for Information Sciences Permanence of Paper for Printed Library Materials, ANSI/NISO Z39.48-1992.

Printed in the United States of America

To my parents, my brother, my sister, and my in-laws

די פּריפעטשיקניקעס: שטענדיק גרייט!
סעלעסטן, מיט אייביקער ליבשאַפֿט
ביילקעןּ, מיכלעןּ, אסתּרלעןּ: וויצן, קינדערלעך, וויצן!
תּם ונשלם שבח לאל בורא עולם

Contents

Acknowledgments   ix

Preface   xi

1 The Most Frequent Procedure   1

2 Visit Time and Clock Time   11

3 What We Want as Patients: Lessons from Communication Science   21

4 The Doctor as a Professional—in Our Eyes   35

5 Measuring How Good Our Doctors Are   51

6 Telling Our Story: Taking the Time to Express Our Health Concerns to Ourselves and Others   63

7 Make the Most of the Visit Through Mindfulness   75

8 How to Communicate Even While Intimidated, Limited, Uncomfortable, or Undereducated   87

9 What We're Talking About: Negotiating the Agenda With the Doctor   101

10 Acknowledge—and Use—Emotion and Motivation   113

11 How to Talk to the Doctor About What Makes You Nervous, Embarrassed, or Grossed Out   127

12 Making Healthy Communities with Healthy Communication   139

13 Learning How to Want Less: Creating a Resource-Sparing Medical Culture Together with Our Doctors   151

14 Transforming Our Health Care System Through Communication and Collaboration   163

Notes	175
Bibliography	187
Index	195

Acknowledgments

My agent, Anne G. Devlin, believed in the importance of this book, and she deserves my gratitude. I look forward to future adventures with her help. Suzanne Staszak-Silva has been a consummate editor, whose direction has immeasurably improved my attempts at clear prose.

My mentors, colleagues, and patients at Bellevue/NYU and Johns Hopkins, as well as at institutions elsewhere and in the wide world of social media, have taught me everything in this book—except for any mistakes, which I will cheerfully correct. I would name names, but then I would forget someone and never forgive myself. To all, then: consider yourself acknowledged, and redeem this acknowledgment for a beverage of your choice the next time we see each other. If you are my patient, I hope that our visits live up to the aspirations in this book.

Preface

The last time you went to your doctor, you might have emerged feeling dissatisfied and disoriented. What did you talk about together, after all? You didn't ask all the questions you wanted answers to, and you don't remember everything the doctor told you. What is the plan? How do we get there? Nothing was clear after you left the office, and you don't know whether it's your fault or the doctor's.

Maybe it's your fault, or the doctor's fault, or the blame can be laid at the feet of the entire health care system. But that's beside the point: the important thing is to identify the problem at the root of this experience and take steps to change it. That's what this book does.

In *Talking to Your Doctor*, you'll learn about the problems with doctor-patient encounters and the difficulties in communication that afflict many different kinds of people. I've observed many thousands of encounters in my job as an internist at the Johns Hopkins Hospital, and use others' fascinating research (together with some of my own) to point the way to a solution: strengthening the doctor-patient relationship through changes in our communication practices and the health care system.

Communicating well with our doctors isn't about being "a good patient," obedient and docile—but it isn't just about being a passionate self-advocate either. Rather, it has to do with being clear about our wishes and expectations and becoming mindful to the complexities of the encounter.

In chapter 1, you'll come along on my eye-opening experiences with doctor-patient communication as a resident doctor in New York City and a new attending physician in Baltimore. You will learn about frequent mistakes we make when we see our doctors and why those encounters are so important—not just for diagnosis or treatment, but to put the doctor-patient relationship on a stable and productive footing.

The minutes set aside for the visit with the doctor will always be limited. But the time in the room where the visit takes place—like the interior of a time-machine—can expand or contract according to the attention that doctor and patient devote to each other. In chapter 2, we will diagram successful and failed encounters between people and their doctors, pointing out what worked and what didn't. Doctor and patient come to the visit with frustrated expectations, outworn grievances, and mismatched experiences, but working on one deceptively simple concept—the conversation—can help overcome these problems and make the encounter productive and health promoting.

Some preparation, both emotional and intellectual calisthenics, can prepare us for rapport with the doctor. Thanks to the new science of doctor-patient communication, the seeds of which were planted thirty years ago, we now understand that communication is not squishy but can be quantified and made rigorous.

In chapter 3, I will explore the sometimes surprising answers that this science offers to the question, "What do we want from our doctor?" and the expectations people have on walking into the visit. We don't always want to make decisions, but we don't want to be talked over either. We will then set the stage for later chapters by talking about how anyone can feel prepared and confident walking in to the doctor's office.

First, we need to think about a topic we're not used to: what our doctors need and want as professionals, and how their conception of their own role needs to change to accommodate the needs of us patients and our society (chapter 4). Then, once we know what we want and our doctors want, we can figure out how to achieve the larger goal: health care that does what's important to us. Is this the same as the "quality health care" everyone is talking about? And how do we define quality after all? Chapter 5 tries to answer that.

The subsequent chapters get into the nitty-gritty of our time in the doctor's office, figuring out how best we can talk about our problems. Chapter 6 helps us prepare ourselves before the visit to understand our own symptoms in a systematic and productive way, making it easier to connect and communicate with the many different people that are part of a usual medical practice.

Chapter 7 introduces mindfulness as a precondition to success in the visit: we need to be emotionally and intellectually ready, centered on the visit and observing every moment.

We might be different from the doctor, and nervous on walking into the room. We might feel limited, intimidated, undereducated, or plain freaked out. Chapter 8 helps us see the visit in a new way: not predominantly as a battlefield to defend our interests, but as a meeting place where, through our shared experiences as human beings, we can find common ground with the doctor to our benefit.

Now we're ready to navigate the visit. We know exactly what we want to talk about and what we need help with—but wait, why does the doctor want to address something completely different? It feels like our agendas are completely incompatible—and they might stay that way until we read in chapter 9 how to negotiate the agenda, a topic that both us and our doctors infrequently address.

Such negotiation is difficult. In fact, the visit with the doctor can be fraught with all sorts of delicate and sensitive emotions: anger, fear, and sadness. Chapter 10 tells us how to confront those emotions and use them to our own benefit in the doctor's visit.

Oftentimes, even if we are ready to communicate, the problems we come to discuss with the doctor stop us in our tracks. They might be gross, impolite, or just things we're not ready to talk about in public, whether they're bowel functions, mental health, or sex. What's the best way to discuss such sensitive issues while not sweeping them under the rug but not being demonstrative about them, either? Chapter 11 will help us through these tricky topics.

By this time we'll have talked a lot about communication with our doctor and how to get the most out of our time with them. Once we leave the doctor's office, however, and get back to real life, there is our community that we're in the middle of. Our health is affected by it, obviously, but we can also make a difference in the health of our surroundings. Chapter 12 reminds us that isolated individuals are not empowered, members of communities are. The principles we have learned in the foregoing chapters—negotiating the agenda and understanding our roles, as well as clarifying our preferences—can help us extend the benefits of communication and a good relationship with our doctor to the other people we live with and among.

The last two chapters lay out a blueprint for remaking our health care system using good communication and productive doctor-patient relationships as a foundation. Chapter 13 talks about the poorly hidden secret more and more people are finding out about: our health care system is afflicted by a severe case of doing too much. Too many tests, too many treatments, and too many studies, none of which are supported by the best scientific evidence, are done in the name of medicine. This overuse doesn't help, but more than that, it can be actively harmful.

Can we remake the health care system to emphasize the relationship between us and our doctor, and encourage good communication practices by us both? I think so, and Chapter 14 outlines how.

Last, the Bibliography (as well as the notes at the end of each chapter) provides sources for further reading and support of my claims. But don't take my word for it: use *Talking to Your Doctor* as a springboard for improved communication with your doctor.

Let me know what you think about this book and your own experiences by emailing zackarysholemberger@gmail.com, leaving a comment at my website, http://zackarysholemberger.com, or visiting the book's site, http://talkingtoyourdoctor.weebly.com. You can also catch up with me on Twitter, @ZackBergerMDPhD, or at the book's Facebook page, http://facebook.com/talkingtoyourdoctor.

Healthy communication to you!
Zackary Berger, MD, PhD

Chapter One

The Most Frequent Procedure

What can we do to improve our health through a workable relationship with our doctor? The answer starts with realizing that doctors can improve their own practice in ways most of them don't even realize. There is a growing science of patient-doctor communication that is underpublicized and underused. It took me a long time to figure out that there was a systematic method to approaching and improving communication between doctors and patients. This process started in medical school.

I never got very excited by discussions of futuristic medical technologies or pharmaceutical innovations. I was always dutiful but less than thrilled in the operating room. The first sense of excitement in my medical education came with the realization that there are as many kinds of patients in the world as people. The lie told about primary care doctors is that, at least in industrialized countries, they see the same kind of diseases over and over again, and their intellect and engagement is lulled by a constant drumbeat of high blood pressure, diabetes, more blood pressure, the occasional case of depression. So why learn this kind of medicine, think the intelligent medical students who want to pay off their loans, especially when the excitement of medicine is in the high-paying and technology-rich specialties?

COMMUNICATION IN THE TEMPLE OF FREE MEDICINE

My initial fascination with medicine had a different source. Instead, I had the good fortune to be stunned by human variety at the temple of public health care and freely provided medicine: Bellevue Hospital in New York City. Patients from everywhere stream through its doors. As a medical student and primary care resident in its clinics, I found myself on the phone with interpreters for languages I had never heard of, let alone heard spoken before. Of course, not every patient was from an exotic locale. Many spoke Spanish and Mandarin. Most spoke English, with the panoply of accents and inflections found in the five boroughs. But there was plenty of Bengali, Tagalog, Wolof, and Cantonese as well.

It was in Bellevue where I realized that every patient, no matter how unique, could be understood with the same set of delicate tools, used for a certain kind of procedure. This realization came to me not by dint of sudden revelation but by teaching and mentorship.

Mack Lipkin Jr., MD, a world-renowned researcher of medical education, doctor-patient communication, and patient-centered medicine, is a professor of medicine at NYU (New York University) Medical Center and director of the residency program at Bellevue Hospital where I trained. He writes in his book *The Patient Interview* that the interview is the procedure most often done by doctors, with the average physician conducting some 150,000 in a lifetime.

Other procedures, like colonoscopies, cardiac catheterizations, and urological surgeries are considered important enough for doctors to carefully hone every movement, to maximize quality and efficiency. Hospitals pour money into the equipment and facilities to support these procedures, and advertise their quality in performing them. In certain widely used hospital rankings, the hospitals' ability to perform such procedures is taken into account. Yet the most common procedure—the doctor-patient interview—has not been perfected quite so carefully, and I have yet to see an advertisement for a doctor or hospital with the tag line, "Best Interview Quality 2013!"

TAKING THE INTERACTION FOR GRANTED

It's easy to take for granted something that's done so often. Dialogues happen so frequently in our interaction with the health care system that they go unrecognized by us. We don't feel well, and talk to our partner or family about it. We decide to contact the doctor's office, where we might have to talk to a receptionist or administrator for an appointment—before we finally manage to get an appointment with the practitioner, be it a physician assistant, nurse practitioner, or physician. Rarely do we think, "How did that interaction go, and how could it have gone better to more effectively pursue these relationships, for the sake of my health?"

As a medical student, I rotated through Bellevue Hospital's alter ego, Tisch Hospital—also a part of the NYU system, but private, English-speaking, and in large part catering to the more advantaged, in comparison to Bellevue's public, Spanish-Mandarin, and sharp-edged raffish nature. In one rotation, I was minding my own business watching an ear-nose-and-throat doctor insert fiber-optic tubes into a patient's nostril. That business over with, the physician asked the patient, without much ceremony, "Do you smoke?" "Yes," said the man. "Well, you should quit," said the doctor. The man had no response.

I thought nothing of this exchange until the physician sat down to dictate his notes. "Patient is an active smoker," he droned. "Smoking cessation counseled." I almost choked on my pencil. Yet at the time—this was almost ten years ago—and even today, there are no legal requirements or even generally accepted professional standards that militate against such a report in the chart. Curtly telling a patient "Stop smoking!" can be reported by a physician as "smoking cessation counseling," no matter how much of a misnomer this is.

Calling this "smoking cessation counseling" is misleading in at least two ways. Counseling requires that advice be given. Advice given preemptorily is more in the nature of a command. Secondly, giving such a "command performance" to an active smoker is effective, but not as effective as counseling, or counseling with the help of medication.[1]

Learning how to talk to a patient is not wasted frippery but improves care. We patients can learn from this as well. If we had had a discussion with our doctor about smoking that was as insufficient and laconic as the one above, what could we have done to make it more productive for us?

HOW BEST TO TALK TO PATIENTS: LEARNING TO LISTEN

In medical school I had an inkling that my peers, and even worse, my mentors, often spoke to patients in the wrong way. It wasn't only that some doctors, the worst of the lot, spoke to patients in a way that I hoped they would never speak to their mother. But it was also that doctors spent an awful lot of time discussing with each other what the best medication might be for a given clinical condition, or the risks and benefits of various surgical procedures, but put precious little thought into telling patients about the medication. "This is for high blood pressure," someone would say, scribbling something illegible on a prescription slip and handing it to the patient. "Take it once daily." "OK," the grandmother would say, putting the piece of paper slowly in her purse without looking at it, as if she would suffer a variety of side effects just by reading the words.

Did the elderly lady know what blood pressure was? How long had she been aware of her diagnosis, and what did she feel about being told she had high blood pressure? What were the options for the treatment of that condition, and the risks and benefits associated with each? What were her preferences, and how much of the decision did she want to be involved in? Finally, even if she wanted the doctor to suggest a treatment to her, what would be possible for her to follow; were there any constraints, financial, emotional, or otherwise that should be made clear when talking about the possible choices? Oftentimes, none of these considerations were discussed—there was just a hurried mumbling of a diagnosis together with the thrust-out prescription slip.

Even though I had this inkling that there might be a better way to talk to patients, I wasn't by any means better than average or immune to these communicative failures. Only after taking note of my own slipups could I begin to think and learn about how good communicators did their job.

One of my first rotations as a medical student was on the obstetrics and gynecology ward, where I conducted checks on dozens of post-partum women at 4:30 in the morning. Bleary eyed but eager to please, we were helpfully furnished with handouts detailing what we should expect on each post-operative day: soon after delivery, for instance, one should be on the lookout for urinary tract infections or blood clots.

But when I went into a room and a sleepless new mother barked at me, peeved at being woken up, "My side hurts!" my first response was to look at the sheet to see if she was "allowed," per the schedule, to have her pain on that day. If it wasn't on the list, I tried gently guiding her into the path that I had there on my paper. "Are you sure you don't have, um, pain when you're urinating?" No, she didn't.

I think the women cut me some slack because I was a medical student and clearly didn't know very much yet. She didn't necessarily want me to fix her symptom but instead to take note of it and bring it to the proper place in the hierarchy so it could be treated by the right doctor. "But you're not hearing me!" one of the new mothers burst out on one occasion, exasperated—which was precisely the problem. It was only during my residency training, in Bellevue Hospital, that I realized how deep the gaps between patient and physician loomed, and how much we could still do to bridge them using the tools that every person on both sides of the dialogue had at their disposal: an ear to hear and a mouth to speak.

It wasn't merely that physicians treated patients inconsiderately; physicians going into the patient's room without an idea how their words would affect the patient was like their going into the ER with only a butter knife and a confident bearing. There was a systematic study to be done, data to be collected, and innovations to be implemented. But how should the doctor go about it? And was there any way to enlist the patients I saw in the improvement of our communication with them? Where was the right place to start?

"WE CAN USE THAT AS DATA"

It started, for me, at a table in the conference room of the primary care residency program at Bellevue. The room was undistinguished and the couches were not plush, but the camaraderie from realizing doctors could care about the way they speak with patients was real.

My memory of Dr. Lipkin at that time can be distilled to one phrase, rendered in a gravelly baritone: "We can use that as data." He said this when we residents, sitting jovially in primary-care fellowship at that table, would talk about our inspiring and frustrating experiences with that day's patients: The patient didn't talk to us at all, but motioned for his wife to speak? We could use that as data. The sick twenty-something was cruel to the secretary and us doctors but sweet as syrup to the nurse? Data. The specialist told the patient that a procedure was obviously necessary, but the patient couldn't tell us why this was so, and no note in the chart had accompanied this determination? More data.

This was a different kind of data: not to quantify and objectify (as is done in randomized controlled trials, thereby to elevate the population without taking into account the unique importance of the individual's circumstances) but to understand and support. Dr. Lipkin, in short, is an expert in how doctors and patients communicate, a gatekeeper to a science that I have begun to practice. As part of our residency, we were required to purchase a heavy blue tome, one of the Springer Verlag scientific works that you never think someone could read cover to cover—but I did, with mounting excitement, paging through *The Patient Interview* as if I had been waiting for it all my life. [2]

One section in particular, on "the difficult patient," drew my attention. You hear that term a lot as a doctor. But instead of complaints and war stories, there was a detailed taxonomy of personalities and their disorders that might explain these behaviors, and information on how best to communicate with such people.

That book and Dr. Lipkin taught us the foundations of understanding doctor-patient communication. We learned about the three functions of the medical interview: gathering information, expressing and dealing with emotion, and managing behavior. These are not static tasks, to be done by rote in the same way with every patient, but are guideposts in the flow of interviews that are ever changing from patient to patient and from visit to visit—whether we are patient or doctor. Dr. Lipkin says, "Each interview provides a fresh beginning"; he means for the doctors in their relationships with the patient. But one could just as well say that each interview provides a fresh beginning for the patient.

If we can use what happens in the interview as data, information for patient and doctor to start afresh with idealistic ends for the sake of health, we can also keep an eye out for common mistakes. Just as parents and children or married couples fall into ruts from which some never recover, so too do doctors and patients often re-enact the same grim dynamic with each visit. We have had visits like this, whether with an unwelcome doctor, boring teacher, a wet blanket of a date, or an oppressive relative. We roll our eyes and immediately tune out.

The doctor feels this way, too. There is no room with less energy than an exam room where doctor and patient can't stand each other. Of course, there are patient-doctor pairs that should be split up for their own good. But there are more that are salvageable. Something good can come even from a doctor and patient who find themselves in a rut. Abandoning their relationship is a mistake. Paying attention to cues is an important start.

THE VISIT WITH OUR DOCTOR: WHAT WORKS, WHAT DOESN'T

In this book we'll talk about what works and what doesn't in our visit with the doctor, whether our goal is better health, a better relationship with our health care provider, or just less frustration when scheduling or experiencing our appointment.

Here's a list to get us started:

- Be alive to opportunities for connection and engagement.
- Be explicit about what should be covered in the visit.
- Be sensitive to topics you find uncomfortable—but try and find ways to maximize your willingness to explore them anyway.

We will also talk about what doesn't work, which is not just the flip side of what does work. If doctors in the past have been more directive and paternalistic than warranted, they should not now fling themselves to the other end of the spectrum and become vague patient-centrists, unwilling or unable to make a decision about what is best for the patient. If doctors have only recently come to realize that medicine should be specific to the individual even in its smallest details, they should not let go of the accompanying truth which is even deeper to medicine: that there is a virtue to experience and systematic knowledge. Sometimes practitioners do know better.

BECOMING INVOLVED IN THE VISIT

By the same token, we must—as patients—become involved in the visit. We are our own best advocates. We know our bodies better than anyone else. The buzzword often attached to these laudable impulses is "empowerment." While there is, traditionally, a significant power imbalance between doctor and patient, we would be wrong to try to "power up" before entering the doctor's office. Indeed, as I will show later, the best communication science shows that when someone tries to "take control" of the situation, that can set back emotional and intellectual cooperation that is at the core of the healing conversation. Some people seem to think that it would be invigorating to exchange perspectives, to move cleanly from physician-centered intransigence and paternalism to patient-centered decision making. But that would be misguided for another reason: not every person is ready or desirous of making significant decisions within the context of the medical relationship. Carl Schneider, PhD, JD, a professor of law and medicine at the University of Michigan, did both doctors and patients a huge favor in his book *The Practice of Autonomy* by summarizing the literature on how often patients really want to be involved in decision making.[3] Although the studies are too different to be summarized in a neat report, we can say that about half of patients want to be involved in a significant way in the decisions they make. If that's true—and more recent science seems to indicate that it is—then patient empowerment must mean something else if it's not to be empty grandstanding on behalf of only the people who are already prepared to make decisions without the benefit of advocacy. Advocating for the patients must be part and parcel of advocating for physicians: we need to be thinking about, and supporting, a relationship that lets both patients and physicians support health in their own way.

When I left the multilingual halls of Bellevue and headed to a dream job at Johns Hopkins, I was confident that the stars were finally aligning on behalf of healthy conversations. This was not just because I had the good luck, in a poor economy, to continue my patient-care experiences at another premiere institution. As I moved to Baltimore and started my new job in the fall of 2009, debate on Barack Obama's Affordable Care Act, known colloquially as Obamacare, was in full swing. In the spring of 2010, the bill was finally passed—despite sturm, drang, and the determined opposition of those who saw the legislation as yet another government takeover of something the private sector should manage.

DOCTOR-PATIENT RELATIONSHIPS: CAN HEALTH REFORM MAKE EVERYTHING BETTER?

I thought that health care reform would begin to make everything better, addressing pressing issues of cost, access, and quality of care. I was about half right. Access, of course, is what the bill is all about—millions will be provided care they would not have gotten before. The cost improvements attendant on the bill are debatable, but nonpartisan estimates indicate that the "cost curve" (the rate of cost increase) might in fact be bent in the right direction over the next few years. Even quality of care is addressed, at least piecemeal, by initiatives written into the bill. One of these initiatives has already emerged from the swamp of legislation, like Venus on the half-shell, with a promising name and charge: the Patient-Centered Outcomes Research Institute.

Patient-Centered! What could be bad about that? And indeed it is very salutary that the concerns of the individual patient are placed front and center in health reform. The closer one looks at what patient-centered outcomes are supposed to mean, however, the less confidence one has that such an initiative has anything to do with a truly healthy conversation between doctor and patient. First of all, "patient-centered outcomes" are meant to be analyzed from a research perspective. Indices will be assembled, validated, and then applied to individual patients. The focus here is not on what an individual patient—you or me—might want, but on what large populations of people tend to want in the aggregate. Even if I want something different, personally, the broader rubric of "patient-centered outcomes" is likely not to include every individual preference.

The healthy conversation we will be talking about in this book is still something, unfortunately, that the current health care system, even in its reformed ObamaCare version, is not promoting intellectually or supporting financially. To understand this point, we need to review the controversy over financial incentives, and how they apply to doctors and patients. Who decides how much doctors get paid, and in turn, how much insurance companies pay doctors—and how much you end up paying the insurance companies? A small group of physicians, meeting behind closed doors under the auspices of the American Medical Association in Chicago, determines payment rates for procedures and visits for Medicare and Medicaid. They are known as the Specialty Society Relative Value Scale Update Committee (RUC). It is a "specialty society" because the committee is made up mostly of specialist physicians—only five spots on the committee are given to primary-care providers. It deals with a "relative value scale" because the committee "updates" the Medicare and Medicaid billing scale, by which most insurance companies operate de facto. The system encourages the incentives that pervert our health care system, favoring procedures over deliberation. Thus it makes perfect sense that the American Academy of Family Practice decided in 2012 to opt out of the RUC and no longer support the relative value scale as it is currently implemented. Many other professional societies, including the Society of General Internal Medicine—of which I am a member—are coming around to their view. (As this book goes to press, revisions to the physician's payment scale are currently working their way through the federal government, but they are currently piecemeal and not in force yet.)

Health care reform, after all, requires not just reform of access—refashioning the health care system so that more people can get care—and quality, but also remaking medicine so that it leads to longer, healthier lives, and fills the unconscionable gaps between rich and poor. It also requires reform of costs. We know that the United States spends more and gets less. Thus, realigning our incentives should make our health care system more efficient. Pay primary care providers more, pay specialists less—any doctor, no matter what their discipline, would recognize this as a sensible goal.

But let's keep our eye on the healthy conversation. Would the doctor-patient relationship, that fragile and neglected foundation, be saved or encouraged by remaking the payment structure? I doubt it. Even if the family practice physicians and general internists manage to put pressure on the RUC to remake the relative value scale—even if procedures are knocked down a peg or two in the payment hierarchy, the upshot will only be that primary care doctors get paid more for the time they spend with patients. Although more time with patients is certainly more valuable than less, what we'll find out in the next chapter is that the clock is only one determinant of the "time dimension" in the exam room.

No payment structure can make doctors and patients understand what their relationship can mean to them. Certainly, primary-care doctors can be paid better, and more minutes on the clock can be scheduled for a given visit. But thirty minutes in the middle of an unsuccessful conversation can feel like six weeks on a desert island with a bad accordion player if the right skills aren't exercised by both parties.

Similarly, we can strive to improve quality, cost, and access in all the top-down ways that science can teach us. As we know, much of the improved lifespan and decreased extent and severity of disease that we have to thank medicine for is not due to the individual art of the doctor as much as to the population science of the public health practitioner. Advocates of health care reform, like me, are confident that support for the best population science applied to our most fragmented and costly of health care systems—this includes the disciplines of health economics, public health, epidemiology, behavior change, and much more—will help people live longer and healthier.

But this leaves out an important piece of the puzzle. Health depends on the individual. There is no effective doctor-patient relationship without the healthy conversation—and that conversation can't be legislated in a top-down way. We need the best science, but that science needs to percolate up from the ground, like dew, not be piped in like irrigation. What follows is an attempt to square the circle, to make you the individual whose unique eyes, ears, and personality will bring the healthy conversation into being: first between two people, then for entire populations. If patient-safety experts now realize that culture always beats strategy, we health communication advocates are coming to this truth only later. Let's make this culture together.

Chapter Two

Visit Time and Clock Time

Imagine your last visit with a doctor. You planned it in advance; it was written on your calendar, with a given number of minutes assigned. You made sure to show up on time, and got impatient if your doctor was late. You might have looked at the wall clock on several occasions. During the visit itself, you might have felt stressed: how were you going to get across everything you had to say in the allotted time?

And when you got home, there are so many things you realized you didn't say to the doctor that you meant to. You had several items on your problem list that you didn't touch at all. You didn't really understand a lot of what the doctor told you, and for the life of you, you can't repeat the advice she gave. It's as if the visit never happened at all, perhaps because everything was compressed into a fifteen- or twenty-minute space.

It's not surprising that many doctors see the length of the visit as an important indicator of its quality. And, by our own experience, we know how important visit time is for us. Isn't it true that we're all dissatisfied with the amount of time we have with the doctor? Isn't it also true that the American health care-system is uniquely hampered by the insufficient time doctors have to spend with patients?

Our intuitions in this area are sharpened by economic pressures. In American health care, we spend more to get less. We are shelling out for more tests and procedures—more MRIs and blood tests—while shortchanging the basic care that matters; we feel this truth so deeply we almost don't need to check whether it's true or not. Thus we would guess that medical visits in the United States are shorter than in other countries.

The length of a visit is indeed an important part of quality health care. As health care communication expert Debra Roter, ScD, a professor at the Johns Hopkins Bloomberg School of Public Health and Judith A. Hall point out,

11

the shorter the visit, the fewer problems identified in the patient-physician dialogue, and the shorter the visit, the less discussion of social or psychological problems with the doctor.[1]

NOT VISIT LENGTH, BUT VISIT QUALITY

However, perhaps these studies are looking at the wrong measurement. It is not the length of the visit per the clock, but the quality of the visit time. If we take a closer look at the intuitions we mentioned above regarding the medical visit—it *must* be shorter than in other places; patients and doctors *must* be dissatisfied with the time allotted—we find that they are not borne out by the facts.

In a landmark study done in the United Kingdom in 1989, the time scheduled for a visit with a primary care doctor was compared with the reactions of doctors and patients to the visit itself, and the actions carried out by doctors as part of the visit. Even in visits scheduled for five minutes, two-thirds of patients felt "very free" to discuss their concerns and 90 percent were very satisfied with the information received.[2] I have never experienced a five-minute visit either as a doctor or patient but cannot imagine being satisfied by so little time.

In comparison to other countries, the time allotted to doctor-patient encounters in the United States is actually longer.[3] Visits in Europe with general practitioners, the equivalent of our primary-care doctors, range from seven to sixteen minutes, with comparable visit lengths in the United States averaging around seventeen minutes. Roter and Hall suggest that the large variability of these set times does not suggest some basic differences in the needs of patients or doctors from country to country—it seems implausible that a foundational dissimilarity between the Dutch and the American psyche, for example, should explain why the average primary-care visit in the Netherlands is ten minutes, while it's seventeen minutes in the United States.

Rather, visit times are an outgrowth of the characteristics of our health care system. This is good news and bad, like so much else about our health care fragmentation: it means that there are no excuses, there is nothing hard-wired about the way things are, but it means that it is all susceptible to change. There is nothing magic about a fifteen or seventeen-minute visit time. We are not stuck with it.

For this reason, we can look beyond the clock. Like another doctor, Dr. Who of the BBC science-fiction television program, we can inhabit a space during our medical visits where time is an elastic dimension, under our complete control. What's lacking during the visit is not clock time, but visit time: quality interactions between doctors and patients that expand minutes beyond their customary dimensions. This explains why we could theoretically feel satisfied after a visit that lasts five minutes, even though it seems implausible. If we have a certain number of concerns, it stands to reason that the likelihood of covering all of them satisfactorily should decrease with less visit time. The fact that our satisfaction could be preserved during a short visit indicates that, apart from covering our problem list, the visit has other functions that can determine its effectiveness.

You've already heard about the three main functions of the medical encounter: to build rapport, exchange information, and discuss possible courses of treatment. Perhaps, though, we need to add a fourth element to this classic list by Mack Lipkin Jr., MD: to stop time. Attention must be paid, mindfulness must be learned and implemented, not just by doctors but by patients, together with their health care providers.

INCREASE VISIT TIME THROUGH MINDFULNESS

Why is mindfulness important? I recall the first thing that Dr. Lipkin taught me about the medical interview: open-endedness. The best way to learn what our true concerns are when coming to the doctor is for the doctor to let us speak our mind fully without interruption. Similarly, for us to communicate optimally with our doctors, we need to let them tell us what they think is important, giving them space to provide their expertise that is not, for the moment, taken up by our complaints. This is a tricky balance: to monitor the flow of the conversation while not forgetting what we want to discuss.

To learn the importance of open-endedness and other qualities of the healthy conversation, we will start by looking at a transcript of a doctor-patient encounter that didn't happen, but could have. Though it's invented, it reflects many aspects of real conversations.

Transcript 1

Ms. Chronic: It's good to see you, Dr. Pressure. I had a terrible time finding parking, though.

Dr. Pressure: Yes, that can happen. How is your blood pressure going? I think that's the real reason for this visit; didn't we agree on that last time?

Ms. Chronic: If you say so, doctor. I am having terrible pain.

Dr. Pressure: We will get to that, but I want to make sure we talk about your blood pressure.

Ms. Chronic: I know when my blood pressure is high. I get these terrible splitting headaches.

Dr. Pressure: Most people can't feel it when their blood pressure is high, unless it's really high.

Ms. Chronic: Oh. I can feel it. It also makes my pain a lot worse [folds her arms, leans back in her chair].

Dr. Pressure: Can you just try to take your high blood pressure pills? It's going to protect your heart.

Ms. Chronic: I take them every single day. I never forget.

Dr. Pressure: Are you sure you never forget?

Ms. Chronic: Maybe once in a while. What should I take for my pain?

Dr. Pressure: Motrin is okay for a couple of weeks, but I worry it can make your pressure worse.

Ms. Chronic: Really? I take it all the time, and I don't feel like my pressure is going high. . . . Doctor, I am really worried there is something going on with my pain.

Dr. Pressure: Um-hm. So here is the prescription for the pressure. Where is the pain?

Ms. Chronic: My lower back. My chest hurts all the time, too. I worry it's my diabetes.

Dr. Pressure: Any urine or bowel incontinence?

Ms. Chronic: No.

Dr. Pressure: Any falls?

Ms. Chronic: No.

Dr. Pressure: It's completely normal, then—sounds like garden-variety lower-back pain. Let me just take a look [starts the physical exam].

Ms. Chronic: Okay. Will you be able to tell me why I feel down? And why I'm forgetting things all the time?

Dr. Pressure: [continues the exam]

In Transcript 1, the doctor starts off the visit by saying, "So you've come in today to talk about your blood pressure." This is probably true—but it's not necessarily the only thing that the patient wants to talk about. Even a half-sentence added to that opening sentence might give the patient a chance to voice her own concern: "I want to talk about your blood pressure today. But what do you want to talk about?"

This is common enough advice and might not be surprising to someone who has been counseled about "self-empowerment" in the doctor's office, or the like. For those who tend toward an adversarial perspective on the doctor-patient encounter, this is something else to ding the doctor on when the satisfaction surveys are filled out.

However, this goes both ways. We have to give the doctor a chance as well. Take another look at Transcript 1, and notice how the patient, once the doctor launches into a hypertension speech, pummels the doctor with a series of her own concerns. She has back pain; her diabetes is worrying her; her chest hurts all the time; she feels down; she thinks she might be forgetting things more often.

None of these concerns are trivial, obviously—they are the very stuff of people's health complaints, and cause great suffering. But even suffering needs to be written down in a list, point by point, and prioritized, otherwise the visit can become entirely subservient to the clock. Which of those problems is bothering her the most? Which did she come to the doctor hoping to talk about? Was there a particular goal that she had for the visit? While it could be that the doctor's poor communication practices kept her from articulating these points, many of us do not take the trouble to come to the doctor with answers to these questions in hand.

By the same token, it is a common thing for doctors to complain about their patients' long lists of complaints that cannot possibly be covered in the space of one visit. While this is true, doctors must be prepared from the outset with a list in hand, or in mind, of what they plan to cover during the visit, with some notion of what is more and less important. Too many doctors treat the items on their list as all of equal importance: either they are going to get through all of them, come hell or high water, or the visit will be a failure. This is unrealistic. Bending a little to allow for negotiation will make it more likely that the most important issues are actually addressed.

Besides the tyranny of time, there is another, more psychological, reason why both patient and doctor need to listen in an open-ended way to the other's concerns. A recent article in the journal *Theoretical Medicine and Bioethics*, by the bioethicist H. M. Evans at the Centre for Medical Humanities in Durham, United Kingdom,[4] talks about an emotion that does not get enough attention in the doctor-patient encounter: wonder. Each person in the room must be prepared to be surprised, on occasion, at what the other has to say, to be shaken out of their own self-centered complaints, becoming ready to work together.

But the doctor and patient can be very different kinds of people. How can doctor and patient be ready to work together and truly listen to each other when each is conditioned, perhaps even trapped, by their own upbringing and environment?

CAN DIFFERENT RACES WORK TOGETHER IN THE EXAMINATION ROOM?

When we think about American health care, which is unequally distributed among black and white, rich and poor, urban and rural, and old and young, we wonder whether some of this inequity might be due to the relationship of doctor and patient. Indeed, Lisa Cooper, MD, Professor of Medicine at the Johns Hopkins School of Medicine and winner of the MacArthur ("Genius") Fellowship, has confirmed just that.

Dr. Cooper is a fascinating and groundbreaking figure—not just in the narrow realm of doctor-patient communication, but in the larger field in which health care inequalities are detected and, we hope, eliminated. In 1999, her article in the *Journal of the American Medical Association* (*JAMA*)[5] confirmed a truth that many people had long suspected. The research question of her paper was this. When African American patients see white doctors, or vice versa, do the patients feel that those doctors take their opinions into account less than if they were of the same race?

We hesitate to bring up the importance of race in the medical encounter, precisely because we know how fraught and important it is. I am a white doctor and most of my patients are African American. My practice is shot through with racial tension. Even if it doesn't come up in every visit, the difference between me and my patients is palpable. I do not think of myself as racist, and certainly most of us don't. But how do we react if we and our doctors are not of the same race?

We must bring up these questions; otherwise we are shutting our eyes to these health inequities. In her 1999 *JAMA* paper, Dr. Cooper found that, indeed, racial discordance predicts a lack of trust in the doctor-patient encounter. She has also begun innovative programs to address health inequality on the basis of this finding—programs whose aim is to improve on a lack of "cultural competence" that might be found among many doctors.

Doesn't this finding mean that my advice about communication might be too general, not applicable to patients of specific groups? If you are African American and your doctor is white, what communication magic is going to bridge that gap? My intuition is that lack of cultural competence, a tendency for the doctor to be out of sync with the patient by reason of ethnic or cultural differences, is not different in kind from general failures of communication. Paying attention to the ways we are talking about things can remedy even cultural and ethnic differences. It could be that different communication techniques are more appropriate to certain kinds of interactions (e.g., if a doctor of a certain kind meets a patient of another kind). But to try and guess what these techniques are would be pure speculation. It might be that patients in one ethnic group are more responsive to statements by doctors that explicitly ask for their opinion, while others might prefer a more directive, "old-school" physician who doesn't.

But for doctor and patient to realize this difference, for us to clearly communicate with the doctor what we are expecting from him or her, requires attention to the other. In other words, both doctor and patient, no matter what kinds of people they are, might do well to exhibit mindfulness.

MINDFULNESS DEFINED: WHAT, WHY, AND HOW—FOR US AND OUR DOCTORS

Mindfulness has been given many different definitions, and I won't dwell here on its connection to Eastern philosophy or religion, such as Buddhism. The most useful definition I know is taken from psychology and the work of Scott Bishop and Mark Lau of the University of Toronto.[6] They propose a two-component model of mindfulness—both components have something to teach the doctor and the patient in the exam room.

The first component is *self-regulated attention*: awareness of one's thoughts and feelings in the present moment. The second component is *orientation*: accepting the continuum of experience. The technical points of these two components aside, I like to think of them in this simplified way: self-regulated attention involves a fine-grained mindfulness of what thoughts and feelings one is currently having, while the orientation to experience involves a "submersion" in the flow. In short, some things can be focused on, while other things can be pushed away. Focus can shift on a nearly continuous basis, depending on how doctor and patient, in their interaction, organize the visit. The engine of the visit is the problems that propel it along from moment to moment. Thus, at any given moment, we and the doctor should be paying attention, in a self-regulated way, to whatever concern is uppermost. However, at the same time, both should be aware of the flow of the visit and not be distracted by individual concerns.

It's best to look at concrete aspects of a sample visit, so let's continue examining Transcript 1. After the doctor's focus on high blood pressure and the patient's recitation of complaints, doctor and patient each stay focused on their own problems. At some point, the doctor begins to direct her attention to the patient's issues, if only by dint of the patient's repetition.

Before they get there, though, the patient goes out of her way to signal that she is not comfortable with the approach to her blood pressure that the doctor would like to take. She says, "Oh," when the doctor points out that her blood pressure is not controlled, according to the doctor's standards. She points out that she takes her blood pressure medication at home "all the time" and that "she would definitely feel it" if her blood pressure were higher. When the doctor asks her how often she takes her blood pressure medication currently, she says, "Every single day. I never forget."

I don't know anyone who never forgets the medication they take. But why would a person not admit to the doctor that she, in fact, does not take her medicine every day as prescribed? There are many reasons: fear of ruining rapport with the provider, shame, denial, and the thought that one will, in fact, as soon as one gets out of the doctor's office, start taking that medication regularly. Just as common, however, on the part of the doctor, is a failure to read the signals that scream, "I worry about the change in blood pressure medications that we are discussing." Or, "I have heard terrible stories about the medication you are talking about. There is no way I am going to take it, but I am not going to be so rude as to say so during this visit."

The reasons a doctor might ignore those signals are also multiple, but illuminating. Providers want to believe that patients are ready to comply; providers worry that assuming patients cannot or will not take the medication as prescribed is tantamount to thinking less of them. Such an assumption is inherent in common language which providers use in talking about the ways in which we do, or don't, take their medication: "compliance," as if medication is a law which we must follow, or "adherence," as if treatment is an unpleasant duty which we must "stick" to, like a poster to a wall. Related language is used to describe us if we do not, for whatever reason, follow suggested therapy: we "deny" that we have forgotten to take our medication, as if we are defending ourselves against an accusation.

Health care providers are not accustomed to listening to objections from their patients. Yes, patients are more empowered these days, thanks in no small measure to the Internet and social media. Everyone can find a community to help them through their illness or medical condition and can bring medical information to the interview that the provider has never seen before. If the provider is not ready to listen, though, even the empowered patient can run up against a wall. And if patients are not ready to listen to the doctor, they can miss the context that renders isolated bits of medical information intelligible or makes clear that a random bit of advice is not something anyone should follow in real life.

THE DANCE OF DOCTOR AND PATIENT: RECOGNIZING THE OTHER'S NEEDS

The solution to the problem of communication is to learn choreography, the dance that doctor and patient must perform together so that communication leads to a healthy conversation. Of course, there is a kind of physical choreography that must matter as well, though the treatment of nonverbal communication lags in the scientific literature. How much might hang on the delicate game of whether a patient prefers the doctor to come out and call him in from the waiting room, or—instead—be placed in the room, waiting for the doctor? Or is there ever a place, in the visit, for the kind of casual nonintimate contact that friends and acquaintances use all the time: a hand on the shoulder, a tap on the knee, a handshake? We know little about this, though Roter and Hall show that such nonverbal communication is not always appreciated.[7]

Here though we are talking about a different kind of choreography, the pas-de-deux of question and response. We navigated this territory in Transcript 1, but in the next chapter we will do it for a visit that "worked" (i.e., with both parties feeling satisfied). The first thing the doctor asks is, "What would you like to talk about on this visit?" This is deceptively simple, and too rarely done.

This is the magic of soliciting the patient's concerns. In my research, based on data from a large, multi-center study of patients with HIV, I learned that doctors often open the visit with general questions about the patient's well-being. In response, patients give general answers.[8] For example, the doctor says, "Everything going all right?" and the patient says, "Fine." There are two ways of understanding this process—that the doctor has used a general formula, a social construction, to lubricate the encounter, and the patient has responded in the same vein. It could also be that the doctor has asked generally how the patient is doing, and the patient has answered that he is, in fact, doing fine—without real complaints.

However, I believe that, most often, doctors and patients understand these opening statements according to the worst of both worlds. This is well expressed by Joanne Lynn and others in their book, *A Handbook for Mortals*, a guide to those facing chronic illness: "When the doctor asks, 'How are you?' and you say, 'Fine,' the doctor thinks he has gathered clinical facts, while you think you've been polite."[9]

I have found in my research that what is "supposed" to happen at the beginning of the visit—the doctor solicits our concerns, and the agenda is built on that basis—does not happen. How can we and our doctors learn to negotiate the agenda? We have to start with all of us recognizing the choreography and then being able to recognize and express our own needs. We will start with our needs as patients, the subject of the next chapter.

Chapter Three

What We Want as Patients: Lessons from Communication Science

I started learning medicine from the poor and sick. They didn't have insurance and often didn't speak English; they had come to America to start a new life and were often stymied by the lack of affordable and universally available medical care. Luckily, there are public hospitals, like Bellevue Hospital in New York, where I did my residency. They patch the holes in our tattered public health system.

There the patients were my most esteemed professors, teaching me that patients are infinitely variable in their response to disease, in the way they approach the physician, and in the interaction between their symptoms, their emotions, and their communication with the doctor. I remember the patient from Peru who told me that his chest pain, which was not related to his heart, felt exactly like an arrow that had pierced his chest and was coming out his back. He was not using a colorful metaphor. He was convinced that an arrow was somewhere inside his body, and it was my job as a doctor to find the projectile. No amount of normal physical exams or imaging could convince him that no such arrow was there. I never found out what caused this pain, but in the final analysis it did not matter. I had to convince myself that his report was correct from his perspective.

Now I am a hospital that is great in a different way. While Johns Hopkins in Baltimore is indeed home to a world-class school of public health, the Johns Hopkins Hospital is not famous for the quality of its primary care. We are a world-class center for doctors in a number of specialties. People come from every corner to obtain the procedure that is not available at home, or to find the source of the pain that has been bedeviling every waking moment. For that reason, I see a number of patients in my practice who come to Hopkins expecting something different there from doctors everywhere else.

This has built up our reputation: Hopkins is where you go to get your internationally renowned specialist of the left nostril, not necessarily the primary care doctor who explains it all to you.

While I think my hospital is one of the best, I think we need to aim at a different kind of excellence. The foundation of all health care everywhere is not just the quality of the procedures but of communication with the patient.

This is not something that people have realized for much of medicine's history. The science of patient-doctor communication is only a few decades old. It is true that, for as long as there have been doctors and patients, there have been much-quoted statements about the importance of paying attention to the patient. William Osler, one of the giants of medical history, the first professor of medicine at Hopkins and one of the founders of medical-student education at the patient's bedside said, "It is much more important to know what sort of a patient has a disease than what sort of disease a patient has." And it actually wasn't even Osler who said this, but Osler quoting some now-forgotten eighteenth-century British physician. It's been a commonplace for more than a hundred years. [1]

Everyone is talking today about patient-centered medicine, and sometimes it is the kind of medicine in Osler's quote that they are referring to. No doctor or patient could quarrel with that statement. The symptom in isolation is not what we care about, and not even the disease by itself. If we are sick we care about our whole body at once, for example, how our high blood pressure interacts with our diabetes, which in turn is affected by sleep problems and depression. Examining any of these problems in isolation is naive at best, dangerous at worst.

WHAT IS REAL "PATIENT-CENTERED CARE"?

Osler could not have foreseen an important achievement of the twentiethth century: a deeper understanding of what "patient-centered care" might actually mean. There are two parts to this understanding. First, we are all authorities about ourselves. Each person knows him- or herself better than anyone else, both body and mind. [2] Caring for people means caring for the whole self, both body and personality.

Second, and even more fundamentally, caring for a patient means understanding that he or she can make decisions completely independent from the doctor. Even when we follow another course of action from the one a medical expert would recommend, the doctor's care should include supporting this decision as long as it is our authentic and final decision.

Thus, a hospital which is world renowned for the excellence of its specialty care should be particularly concerned with doctor-patient relationships. Someone must take care that neither patient nor doctor be lost in the maze of tests and referrals that can come with the workup of a disease. Someone must have the wholeness of the sick person at heart.

So, if at Bellevue I learned to communicate with patients from every continent and (with the help of a translator) in every language, at Hopkins I have learned to appreciate the choice that everyone must make between their own self-knowledge and another's expertise.

DIFFERENT PATIENTS, DIFFERENT DOCTORS

Given the differences between the hospitals, you might also think that there are differences among the people that go to them. You would be right. Baltimore is not New York. In Baltimore there are fewer immigrants. There are Spanish speakers, but not as many as I had in my practice at Bellevue. There are Chinese speakers, but instead of people fresh from Fujian province in China in their first apartments on the Lower East Side, they are graduate students on the way to one of the graduate schools at Hopkins. Most important is Baltimore's status as a city whose population is mostly African American.[3]

New York is shades of brown, Baltimore is black and white. Does this mean doctors need to speak to us differently depending on where we live? What if you are a patient who doesn't fit into the majority where you are, for example, a black person in a majority white city or vice versa? Or someone without much money in a relatively wealthy area? How can you be sure that your concerns are heard, so that you and the doctor can participate in a conversation whose center is your health?

There are differences among us, and these differences can definitely affect the way we talk to our doctors, but there are also deep and universal similarities. Some of these are intuitive: we want to be listened to, we want our concerns heard, we want to feel better, and we want to stay healthy. But not all of them are. Some of them need to be discovered by science. Over the past few decades, the science of patient-doctor communication, something Sir William Osler never knew about, has come about. Some of its findings are what I will detail in this book, and what will help prepare you to bring a healing conversation to your time with the doctor.

COMMUNICATION SCIENCE FOR THE BENEFIT OF PATIENTS: A BRIEF HISTORY

There are many ways to approach the history of doctor-patient communication. One is through the history of medicine. In an article in the *International Journal of Surgery* in 2007, R. Kaba, a surgeon in London, and P. Sooniaku-maran ably traced the development of the doctor-patient relationship throughout time. Kaba quotes a historian who says that the view of the patient in any given period is dependent on that period's view of disease.[4] Thus, for the Egyptians, their doctors were priests, and the patient approached them with awe, as a worshiper comes to a temple. For the Greeks, the physicians were adherents of a logical philosophy, and the patient was part of an experiment in health. And so on. Only with the success of the physical and biological sciences in the twentieth century did paternalism—benevolent condescension toward the patient—become the norm. If medicine is science, then it should be left to scientists. Who asks the beakers in a chemistry lab how they feel?

That is an interesting theory but only goes so far. History does not entirely explain how we act when we are sick. We should approach our doctor with an understanding of how we act when we're affected by that particular illness. I have met a number of patients who say to me, "I know my own body." You can understand this as a way of calling attention—legitimately—to yourself in the visit with the doctor. But I think we all, when we go to our doctors, should talk about our bodies specifically, without shame. We should use phrases like, "I am a person whose throat gets really painful when I have a cold, I always worry I am going to die from an infection." Or, "I think I am going to die early from heart disease, like my uncle did. Whenever I feel a pain in my chest I am reminded of this."

Nonetheless, doctor-patient communication is certainly affected by the characteristics of contemporary society. Just as biomedicine today spends too much to accomplish too little, communication between doctor and patient is today too focused on information transfer and too little on personal connection. That is the best way to understand the history of doctor-patient communication science: not as a steady evolution through various forms of society or scientific understanding, but as a regular returning, in fits-and-starts, to what most of us know to be true about the relationship between doctor and patient.

And what do we know to be true? When we go to the doctor, we want to be listened to. We want to interact with a person who cares. We want to form a relationship. But by the same token, we want someone knowledgeable and competent. We want to leave satisfied and feeling better.

Why then do we find it so difficult to ensure that these things happen when we see the doctor? Why do we feel like we are not listened to? Why does the doctor seem like a hurried automaton and not like a caring person? Why do we never feel like we are in a caring partnership? And, finally, even when we do feel that the doctor is competent in his or her profession, why do we leave unsatisfied, as if our true concerns are not being met?

There are systematic reasons why these things are happening that have to do with the characteristics of the hospital or clinic, and certainly with our fragmentary health care system. We will address these later. There are also doctors who have problems interacting even on a basic human level and have problems that this book cannot address. However, we will assume that the majority of our doctors are people of good will and want to do well by us. We will not subscribe to any conspiracy theories about the medical-industrial complex.

WHAT'S LACKING IN OUR DOCTOR-PATIENT RELATIONSHIPS

So why the gap between us and our doctors? It has to do with the fine details, the aspects that make every interaction unique. This is where the doctor-patient relationship comes in.

There are a number of important basic understandings of this relationship that I should describe. Several of them have become known by the names of their discoverers or practitioners. If you have not heard of these developments, you should, because they might offer practical routes to improve communication with your doctor, even before we talk about the details of the communication science.

Michael Balint was a Hungarian-born psychoanalyst. He was an advocate, among others, of the focal psychotherapy school, in which one specific problem chosen by the patient is the focus of interpretation. He and his coworkers said that "To our minds, an 'independent discovery' by the patient has the greatest dynamic power."[5] How do a psychotherapist's theories relate to medical care? During the final years of his career, Balint supported the creation of "Balint groups," for doctors to discuss psychodynamic factors in relation to patients—that is, any one of us who approaches a health care professional for mental or physical care.

Balint groups are now *de rigueur* in training programs that recognize that we all have barriers in our lives that make healing difficult. These groups provide opportunities for doctors to discuss their patients for whom they feel unable to provide the best care.[6] In other words, Balint groups are the forerunners of today's support groups for patients, with one important difference.

Patient support groups usually focus on the problems faced when confronting disease. Diabetics help each other; people with chronic pain advise each other on how to make that pain bearable. In such groups, we also discuss how to navigate a forbidding health care system. But what these groups don't do is specifically discuss our communication difficulties with our doctors and how to overcome them in a relationship-based way.

Yes, there are plenty of advice-givers who tell us to march into our doctors' offices with a take-charge and confrontational attitude. This might work for some doctors, who might be surprised to find out that you have opinions of your own about your health care. But, as I will discuss further in later chapters, health care is based first of all on a relationship. Why not create Balint groups where we can discuss why we don't get along with our doctors, and think about solutions to these personal incompatibilties? Far better, in some cases, to rework a mismatched doctor-patient relationship than to choose a new doctor.

A SUPPORT GROUP FOR PATIENTS

Imagine for a moment that you are part of such a group, which we could call a "Balint Group for Ordinary People." You have gathered in a room with a diverse group of individuals who have one thing in common: they are currently seeing doctors or other health care providers, or they have occasion to be seen in a hospital. You speak up:

> "I saw Dr. Martin, and she was fine, but I wonder if I am getting on her nerves. Plus, whenever I bring up a problem, she seems like she doesn't know what she's talking about. How can I make her feel like I am paying attention, and want to have a grasp of details, without insulting her or making her feel like I don't trust her?"

Another member of the group pipes up.

> "Here is a way that worked for me. I tell her that I have an interest in knowing what the medical literature says, because I want to do my own research. That way, she has an out to send you whatever pieces of literature she may think are relevant to your question. At the same time, she will be able to learn some things on the topic you are worried about."

Let's create such communities in our own homes, supplemental to but not supplanting other kinds of support groups. We are not working against our doctors but with them. They have emotional and relationship needs as well, and we can build strategies to bridge the gap with them.

THE DOCTOR'S ROLE AS GATEKEEPER

Another pioneer in understanding the relationship between us and our doctors, and an essential step for us to acquaint ourselves with the current science of doctor-patient communication, is the work of Talcott Parsons. Parsons's work is summarized by the medical sociologist James J. Hughes in his "Organization and Information at the Bedside"[7] as the first to theorize the doctor-patient relationship. His approach is called *functionalist*. According to this understanding, patients act a certain way toward doctors, and vice versa, because we are each filling certain roles in society.

We go to doctors because they are the gatekeepers to society's definition of "sick." We cannot, for example, take off work or get benefits due the sick person without the doctor's say-so. As frustrating as this conception might seem, and as limiting, we can use it to our benefit as patients, just as we put the concept of the Balint Group to work. As opposed to this older understanding of the functions of the patient and the doctor, we can say that both play different roles today: as parties to a collaborative relationship. This relationship is reciprocal. The patient's role is to give the doctor an opportunity to heal, and the doctor's role is to make sure that patients have an opportunity for full partnership.

The last preliminary figure we will meet in the history of doctor-patient communication research is Thomas Szasz, a psychiatrist who published a ground-breaking paper in 1958 in the *American Journal of Psychiatry* with his collaborators Marc Hollender, a psychiatrist known for his work on sexual behavior, and William F. Knoff.[8]

TYPES OF DOCTOR-PATIENT RELATIONSHIPS

Szasz, Knoff and Hollender's approach is composed of two parts. First is a historical skepticism. They examine the doctor-patient relationship in the context of various historical epochs, like the article by Kaba and Sooniaku-maran we discussed earlier, and come to the conclusion that "the cultural relativity of the doctor-patient relationship should make us skeptical of the assumption that our current practices are 'good' or the 'best possible.' Probably more often than not, they are neither, but simply reflect the congruence of social expectations and socially shared ethical orientations of physicians." This is paradoxically freeing. If we are not aspiring to some unattainable ideal, trying to find the perfect doctor to end all doctors, we can make a healing relationship with our doctor even within our cultural and historical constraints.

The other important contribution of Szasz and Hollander, for which they are most often cited, is their classification of types of doctor-patient relationship related to different types of illness. When we are acutely ill, according to this theory, we are more passive, yielding absolutely to the doctor's directions. When the doctor is administering a particular treatment, for example a vaccine, the relationship with them is characterized by cooperation toward a given end. Only in chronic diseases do the patient and doctor work together with "mutuality," in which the goals are determined together.[9]

A current version of this outlook, by Stewart and Roter, lays out four different kinds of doctor-patient relationship, each characterized by a different perspective: the paternalistic (in which the doctor exercises control), the consumerist (in which the patient exercises control), the default (in which neither party exercises control) and mutuality, in which both parties work together. [10]

The weaknesses of these classifications limit their usefulness for us when we see doctors. First, they are heavily influenced by psychological theory. There is nothing wrong with a psychological understanding of the doctor-patient relationship (and we will return to such an understanding many times in this book), but like much in psychology, which explains behavior through the dynamics of personalities, we are not left with practical direction about how to change matters to our advantage, or to promote our health. Psychology is not destiny.

Second, these categories are presented as mutually exclusive boxes—but we all know doctors who are at times controlling, at times generously allowing for the development of a healthy relationship. Finally, these psychological approaches are more suited to a medical visit where one sort of thing happens (for example, someone's visit to a therapist) than the medical visit where multiple activities might be carried out, such as discussion, examination, and decision.

Even if we grant, for the sake of argument, that these psychological views of the doctor-patient relationship are set in stone, and indeed analyses do show that we see our relationship with doctors as either patient-controlled or doctor-controlled, [11] it doesn't follow that a psychological approach to our relationship with our doctor will guarantee better care. Yes, much of the current literature on doctor-patient communication focuses on these psychological categories, but perhaps what we have here is a mere repetition of theoretical dogma. Maybe what we should do instead, more practically, is dissect the medical visit into its constituent parts. Unlike in a visit with the therapist, there are a number of moving components to one's visit with a medical doctor.

DISSECTING OUR VISIT WITH THE DOCTOR

Usually, these moving parts are called the history, the physical exam, and patient education and counseling, although there are some more parts that are just as important and often overlooked. Each part of the visit has been examined by communication science, bringing empirical observation to bear where theory can be inexact and unhelpful. And each part demands different things from us to get the most out of our relationship with the doctor.

Here are the parts of the visit as I see them:

1. Introduction/Meeting
2. Agenda Setting
3. Patient's Concern

4. Physician's Response
5. Dialogue and History
6. Physical Exam
7. Discussion of Testing/Information Provision
8. Education and Counseling
9. Closing Exchange

If you think about all these parts before you go to the doctor, you might become overwhelmed. But think again. Most of these are just social conventions, formulas that we and our doctors use. You have used such formulas in countless other social situations, so there's no reason to think you can't learn them in the service of a good relationship with your doctor.

Introduction/Meeting: At the introduction to your doctor, your first meeting with them, you will find out what sort of person they are: their sex, their race, gender, or ethnicity, their age, and what they look like. You shouldn't be surprised to find out that these things matter quite a lot to the doctor-patient relationship. When the doctor is a woman, visits last longer, have more psychosocial talk—discussion about emotions and family difficulties, for example—is shared, and the visit as a whole is more patient centered. [12]

The sensitive issue of race is also important in meeting your doctor. Relationships that are race-discordant (i.e., in which you and your doctor are of different races) are associated with poorer communication. [13] While this has been known for some time, a new study in the *American Journal of Public Health* looked at the effect of a doctor's implicit racial bias, using a test called the Implicit Association Test, on ratings of care by their patients. Black patients reported lower satisfaction and poorer communication from physicians who were shown to have higher levels of implicit bias, according to that test. [14]

This finding is not surprising, and the study is not airtight; for example, the patient's report about the visit was made about nine months after the doctor completed the bias survey. But it lends credence to what some of us have had a sinking feeling about for a long time: our doctors share some of the fallibilities of human beings, racism among them. Not high-grade hate-crime racism, but implicit racial bias, which the physician might not even be aware of.

Thus seeing your doctor face to face might be significant in predicting how you might relate to him or her. (And we haven't even talked about the doctor's style of dress or how he or she greets you.) But does such prediction really matter? Often we are locked into health plans, or for other reasons either practical, logistical, or financial we don't have complete control over who sees us in the doctor's office. Perhaps, though, armed with this information, we can try to address issues of race and gender up front.

Once you have made in into the room and met the doctor, either for the first time or for a return visit, it is time to discuss what the visit is going to be about. Such agenda-setting might be natural to you in meetings with other professionals, but it doesn't come naturally to all of us. Chapter 9 will go into such agenda-setting in detail.

Part of setting the agenda has to do with how we express our concern to the doctor. Telling the doctor about a concern is not just a simple matter of describing it. Any presentation of a problem can hide assumptions about what we think is going on and what we want to do about it. For example, if we say "I am having a cold," then—most likely—the doctor will assume we have a cold. There is nothing wrong with that if we are suffering from an open-and-shut case of upper respiratory infection due to a virus. But what if we are afraid it is something worse? What if we have never felt this way and are sure we are coming down with a real pneumonia? What if we are on medicines that suppress our immune system, and we know for a fact that we should be super vigilant about every symptom? Saying that we are having a cold is the wrong way to start matters off. Of course, we could say that it is the doctor's job to look beneath the surface and figure out what the real reason is behind our "cold," but doctors are fallible and jump to conclusions just as we do. [15]

Another reason to be careful in the presentation of our concern is that the very method of our presentation, beyond what the doctor thinks the diagnosis might be, can determine our treatment options. Let's take two examples.

Example A

> You: Doctor, I am really concerned about prostate cancer. I would like to know how to prevent it.

> Doctor: Well, let's discuss how and whether to get the PSA blood test.

> You: What is that?

[Ideally, you and the doctor would then discuss the pros and cons of the controversial prostate cancer blood test.]

Example B

> You: Doctor, I am really concerned about prostate cancer. Can we discuss what the options are?

> Doctor: Well, it's an interesting thing about prostate cancer. One out of six men are diagnosed in their lifetime with prostate cancer, but the lifetime risk of death from prostate cancer is only 2 percent. [16] Sometimes,

doing nothing is the best option when it comes to screening for prostate cancer.

You: I'm not sure I am comfortable with doing nothing.

Doctor: OK, let's discuss the options then.

Do you see the difference between Example A and Example B? If, for example, you had thought about prostate cancer, knew that it tends not to kill people, and came to the conclusion that doing blood tests for the condition might do more harm than good (since a biopsy can lead to urinary, sexual, and bowel problems)—then you might come to the conclusion that doing nothing is your choice. However, if you came in presenting your concerns as in Example A, you might put yourself on the path to having a biopsy just because your worry about cancer was uppermost. Communication between you and your doctor is also affected by your preferences.

Setting your agenda, and making your concerns known, has been much discussed in recent medical articles. The importance of identifying your preferences is clearly important, not just in regard to end-of-life decision making[17] (where the body of literature is probably the greatest) but about all medical conditions, especially chronic conditions like diabetes[18] or hypertension[19] for which there are many different options for treatment, but often not clear evidence about which choice is better than another.

IDENTIFYING PREFERENCES—OR MAKING DECISIONS?

Even though identifying preferences is important, and doing so seems to lead to better care, this doesn't mean that it's easy to do. This difficulty is due to many factors, but predominant among them is confusion between *participating in the decision process* and *shared decision making*.

As many people know, recent decades have seen a shift in how doctors are taught to relate to us. Paternalism, in which we are talked down to as a parent to a child, is now frowned upon. Patient-centered care is now the reigning paradigm.

Unfortunately, it's not clear what patient-centered care means in the modern age. Many people have assumed that this is the same thing as shared decision making, in which the patient and the doctor sit down together and, for instance, decide what medicine to use for high blood pressure. There are two problems with this assumption, however. First, the physician's goals are not always your goals. As a result, it has been suggested recently that we need to clarify what our own goals are as patients when we go to the doctor—and those should be the aims of our medical care.[20]

But even if we clarify our own goals, it doesn't follow that we need or want to share in the decision that the doctor makes. Sometimes we want more information than what the doctor is giving us, sometimes we want to take part in the decision, and sometimes we want neither. In a classic article in the *Journal of the American Medical Association* in 1984, Willliam Strull and co-authors found that "clinicians *underestimate* patients' desire for information and discussion but *overestimate* patients' desire to make decisions."[21]

Thus what we need to do, not just as part of setting the agenda but throughout the visit, is make clear to the doctor how much we want to participate in the process. Do we want the doctor to decide, in general? Do we want to be involved in the details of the process? Both these ends of the spectrum are fine, but they should be made clear up front. I can't yet point to any scientific article proving that this leads to better health or greater satisfaction for us when we go to the doctor, but it's clearly the next logical step.

We have moved from assuming that the doctors should make all decisions; to realizing that doctors and patients both have a voice; to (mistakenly) assuming that patients should make a decision together with physicians in all cases. Our next move should be to clarify how we want to be involved in the process. An example might go like this:

Patient: It feels like there are a number of alternatives here.

Doctor: That's right. There's no 100 percent answer.

Patient: I am pretty comfortable doing what you want, Doctor, but I need to let you know that I don't like medicines.

Doctor: That's helpful. Thanks.

What about the parts of the visit that come after agenda setting and identifying our concerns? The history and physical exam are also important for us and the doctor. When the doctor starts to ask you about your symptoms, or he is starting the physical exam, there is one piece of advice to give that many have given before: ask questions. The medical history is not a one-way arrow where we feed information into the doctor's computer. We can ask, for example, "Why are you asking me that question? I wonder if you are asking me these things because . . . ." The same holds true for the other parts of the visit, for example, where the doctor informs and counsels you. Stewart and Roter found that only 6 percent of statements in doctor-patient visits are patient questions—perhaps out of a mistaken sense that questions are inappropriate.[22] But they are always appropriate.

I've talked a lot in this chapter about how we all can clarify our preferences in the doctor's office—not about what antibiotic a doctor wants to give (most of us aren't interested in assuming responsibility for that level of detail), but about what part we all want to play in decision making. In other words, are we hands-off or hands on?

However, such expression of preferences might be intimidating for us to handle, especially if (like me) we are naturally intimidated, ill-at-ease, or uncomfortable when going to the doctor. How do we muster up the confidence to make this happen? Do we need to be militant, take-charge, confrontational types, born patient advocates? No. We just need to do what we do every day—understand the person across the table from us and actively communicate.

In the next chapter, we will start by understanding what the typical doctor might want from us, and use that as one of our basic building blocks in constructing a healthy relationship.

Chapter Four

The Doctor as a Professional—in Our Eyes

THE DOCTOR IS IN—BUT SOMETIMES, UNCERTAIN

I have a confession to make. I am a doctor who doesn't know everything. You come into the room to see me, and I am not sure if we are really addressing your chief concerns. When you tell me your story, I am not 100 percent certain that we have gotten all the details we need. Perhaps there are things you haven't divulged because you think there isn't enough time, you are embarrassed, or you think that I think they aren't important.

After I get the details of your history, I start in on the physical exam. I check your blood pressure. (You say that the medical assistants checked it once out in the hall before the visit already? True, but we can't be sure that they checked it after giving you five or ten minutes to rest, per the best guidelines for checking blood pressure.) It is high. I am not sure if this is your true blood pressure. I know that you are in pain today, and pain raises blood pressure. I could order a twenty-four-hour blood pressure check with a monitor that you wear, but I need to think about that.

After I check your blood pressure, I look at your hands, feel your pulse, and feel the pulse in your neck. I listen to your heart and lungs. I look in your throat and have you swallow so I can feel your thyroid. I feel, listen to, and tap your abdomen. I look at your legs. I check your reflexes with the hammer. If you have diabetes or have other problems with the sensations in your feet, I might check the soles of your feet with a thin wire.

Every part of the medical history and physical exam, and every answer you give, every question I ask and body part I examine is a kind of test that gives me information. Unfortunately, these tests are fallible. And, even if the information they gave me were perfect, I am also fallible. After the welcome, discussion of your concerns, agenda setting, history review, and physical exam, I have a pile of information that I am not sure how to synthesize into a treatment plan. This is not because I am a worse doctor than average. I am confident in my abilities and pretty good at what I do. Nor is it because of my medical specialty, though the stereotype about us internal medicine doctors is that we think too much. No, I think that all doctors, no matter what their specialty, are confronted by this uncertainty throughout the visit. Indeed, the well-known surgeon and medical writer, Atul Gawande of Harvard University, wrote an entire book about such uncertainty. [1]

We don't acknowledge this uncertainty to ourselves or our colleagues, or—most important—discuss it with our patients. There are many reasons that keeping our uncertainty under wraps is not a tenable situation. First is safety: everything we do as doctors involves some risk, and not revealing our uncertainty means that you have a misleading idea of the risk-benefit balance for a given suggested treatment.

The second reason has to do with the general medical culture. People go to doctors for an assurance that all will be well, that there is an expert out there who can make everything better. They see the doctor as previous generations saw the priest. [2] We all, at certain junctures, wish to place our fate in the hands of someone else. There is nothing wrong with letting a physician serve certain pastoral functions, tending to our spiritual as well as our medical needs. But that does not require the doctor to wear a mask of infallibility.

This leads to the third reason doctors should be open with you about what they know and don't know: honesty. A relationship should have that quality. From an everyday perspective, if there were someone you went to regularly for advice about practical matters, wouldn't you like to hear from that friend if they had no idea what answer to give? Or if they felt as though their experience or knowledge was simply insufficient to answer your question? How much more should a doctor be prepared to tell you that they don't know.

WHAT DO DOCTORS NEED AND WANT?

We should take pity on our doctors, whose difficult situation is not sufficiently realized. Our culture is now rightly suspicious of a bygone culture in which doctors did not listen to the patient. However, as a reaction to the excesses of patriarchal medicine, we don't think about what doctors need or want. Take, for example, the recent controversies over the usefulness of screening tests for prostate cancer.

The risk for a man of dying from prostate cancer sometime in his lifetime is about 2–3 percent. However, a study of healthy organ donors between 1994 and 2000 who were autopsied after dying suddenly revealed that half of men between 70 and 80 years old harbored hidden, or occult, prostate cancer, but it wasn't the cancer that killed them.[3] Add to this the fact that biopsying the prostate (taking a piece of it in a surgical procedure to see whether there is any cancer growing within it) is not without risks. Even if the biopsy proceeds without complication, there is a danger that the patient could have problems afterward like urinary or stool incontinence or erectile dysfunction.

Or take the case of mammography. Recently, the United States Preventive Services Task Force recommended that mammograms be done every two years for women over fifty. However, for women younger than fifty, "clinicians may provide this service to selected patients depending on individual circumstances"—but in the majority of cases, the benefit is likely to be small.[4] Not a simple discussion, either if we are expecting a mammography or if our doctor decides we are "select."

The doctors are supposed to have evidence at their disposal and come to patients with a set of options. What are they supposed to do, though, if the options themselves are not clearly delineated? A mammogram can be done every two years. For some women, there might be some evidence that it can be done less often.[5] To take yet another example, a bone mineral scan, or DEXA scan, is supposed to be done at least once after menopause in order to catch low bone density and thereby prevent fractures. However, it's not clear how often it should be done again after that one time, if at all.[6]

All these situations, in which there is no certain answer, put the doctor in a difficult position. To understand why this is, we need to define what we expect from the doctor, and what doctors expect from themselves. The term used for this nowadays among doctors is "professionalism." There are expectations of doctors that would be considered above and beyond, even morally superior, in an ordinary person: the expectations of long and sometimes tedious training, of attending to a patient even at inconvenience or risk to themselves. As we compare various statements of professionalism, requirements and expectations for doctors, to what they actually think their own role should be, we will find interesting gaps and differences. For that matter, what we think doctors should be doing does not always fit with what is stated by their own professional organizations.

CONCEPTS OF PROFESSIONALISM: FROM GREECE TO TODAY

We could find a worse place to start than the Hippocratic Oath. This oath was written in the fifth century, BC, in Greek, and is characterized both in form and content by a number of formulas: an appeal to the gods, a list of specific items to which the oath-taker is swearing, and finally a section detailing what might happen to the oath-taker if any of the promises are broken.

We might think that a religious formula from a polytheistic society written more than two thousand years ago has little to teach us today. Not entirely, though. The oath-taker says that he will "impart a knowledge of this art to my own sons, and to my teacher's sons, and to disciples bound by an indenture and oath according to the medical laws, and no others."[7] There's a guild system that still partially characterizes medicine. There are bars to entry and little incentive to lower them. Thus, only a certain slice of society, the slice that can afford astronomical tuition and overcome the not inconsiderable social barriers to the profession, is allowed into medical school. An even slimmer slice manages to stay in, finish, complete residency, and make it into the ranks of active doctors.

Next, the oath-taker says that he will "prescribe regimens for the good of my patients according to my ability and my judgment and never do harm to anyone. . . . I will give no deadly medicine to anyone if asked . . . I will preserve the purity of my life and my arts." In any house into which the oath-taker comes, he will enter only for the good of his patients.

These are moral claims. The physician sets him- or herself apart from ordinary people. Note that little is said here about how much the physician knows. Knowledge does not enter into this concept of the physician's job. Rather, his or her ability and judgment are key.

These qualities can be intuitively attractive to us as patients. We would like doctors to realize that they don't know everything. Their skill lies in judgment and their ability to explain matters to us so that they can help us make our own decisions. On the other hand, contrary to the Oath, some of us expect our doctors to have a store of knowledge.

What do doctors want to be? How do they see themselves? Do they think ability and judgment, or store of knowledge, is more important? How do these two views affect our view of doctors, and can the two views be bridged in a realistic conception of the role of the doctor?

Ideally, there would be a survey about what doctors think about themselves and the contradictions between their professional standards, society's expectations, what we patients want from them, and the compromises of real life. There is something like such a survey, which was done by Eric Campbell and co-authors at Massachusetts General Hospital several years ago.[8] They asked doctors how much they agree with so-called norms of professionalism, (i.e., the ideals that many groups of doctors have agreed to, and to what extent their behavior actually conforms to these ideals).

WHAT DOCTORS THINK ABOUT NORMS OF PROFESSIONALISM: TWO STUDIES

The survey is interesting as much for what it doesn't show as for what it does. The survey polled 1,662 physicians, and 58 percent of them responded, which reminds you that a survey is only as good as who answers it. We won't know if the doctors who didn't answer are the ones we don't like—because they don't care about standards of professionalism—or the ones we do—because they are too busy taking great care of their patients.

Campbell, et al., set out to discover how much of a gap exists between what doctors believe, whether in the Hippocratic Oath or in the new ethical guidelines of the American College of Physicians, and what they do. Most doctors agreed with uncontroversial statements that might be found in professionalism standards. For example, the great majority agreed that "physicians should minimize disparities in care due to patient race or gender." Ninety-six percent of those who responded also agreed that doctors should report impaired or incompetent colleagues to the relevant authorities. However, what doctors agreed with was not always what they reported doing. For example, 45 percent of respondents said they had not reported such impaired or incompetent colleagues.

You can understand this study in two ways. The first is optimistic: doctors agree to things they are by and large supposed to agree to. They want to treat us equally without regard to gender or race; they know to report colleagues with problems to the right authorities; they want to improve professionally. Perhaps we are not surprised. When we take surveys, we might not say things that we would divulge only to our closest friends. But at the very least, it is reassuring to hear that what doctors say in the context of a research study fits with what we would like them to say.

The pessimistic reading of these results is that, when the rubber meets the road, doctors do not always do what most people think is necessary. Is this because the doctors do not truly agree with the statements they endorsed in the survey? Because their systems are not set up to make doing the right thing actually possible? Or is it because there are too many competing priorities?

Such a gap between the ideal and the real, or between formal statements of professionalism and the actual everyday experience of doctors, reminds us of the limits of research. We can ask doctors what they do or don't do, but perhaps we need to do it in a more informal setting, where they feel free to talk about what really happens and why. This requires a different kind of research method, called "qualitative research." This term itself includes various kinds of research methods, but it goes by this name to distinguish it from studies which, on the basis of statistics, try to isolate statistical relationships between individual variables defined in isolation. Qualitative research, on the other hand, is more exploratory, and is used to define the problem and help specify an approach when we don't know what relationships to examine in more detail.

Such a study was conducted by P. Wagner and colleagues at the Medical College of Georgia.[9] Like the study I mentioned earlier, and like any scientific study, the gaps in their findings will tell us as much about what we should learn from their study as their results themselves. Wagner and co-authors start with the assumption that the principles of professionalism are more or less agreed to: "commitments to professional competence, honesty with patients, patient confidentiality, maintaining appropriate relations with patients, improving quality of care, improving access to care, just distribution of finite resources, scientific knowledge, maintaining trust by managing conflicts of interest and professional responsibilities." Let's accept their assumption for now, though the authors admit, with refreshing honesty, that not everyone agrees with this list. Also, I think some items might have been left off, if only because of the incompleteness of current professionalism guidelines: What about being a healer? What about making sure that patients feel better, or at least satisfied, after walking out of the room? Not everyone would agree that these requirements are included under the dry term "professional competence."

The authors interviewed attending physicians, medical students, and even everyday people (i.e., patients) to find out how they understood "professionalism" differently. Unsurprisingly, certain themes were common among all groups: attending physicians, residents (junior doctors) and patients. The main themes understood to be part of professionalism were technical skills, relationship with the patient, and "character virtues" (i.e., being of good character). Other themes which were common to all groups included the uniqueness of medicine as a profession, congruence between personal characteristics and behavior, and the importance of relationships with one's colleagues.

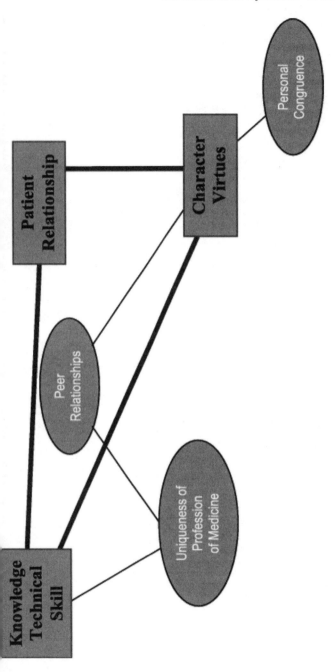

Figure 4.1. Basic professionalism map.

There were some enlightening differences between groups, however.

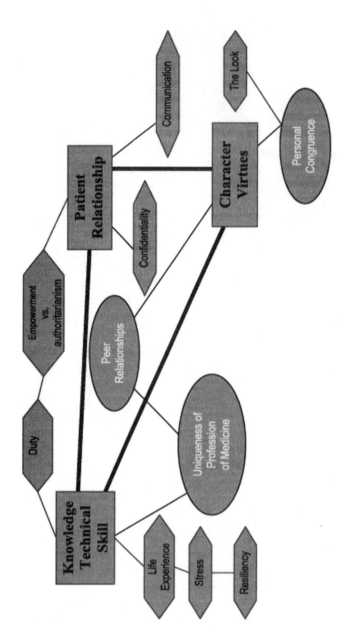

Figure 4.2.   Faculty professionalism map.

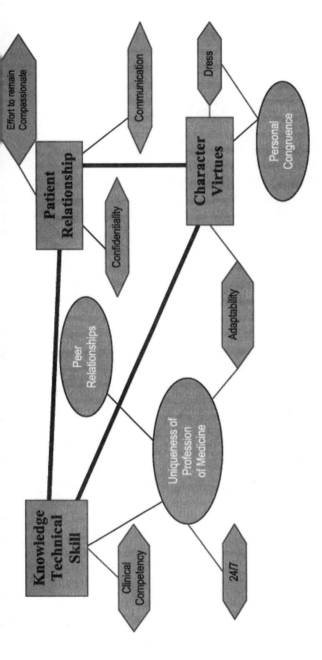

Figure 4.3.   Resident professionalism map.

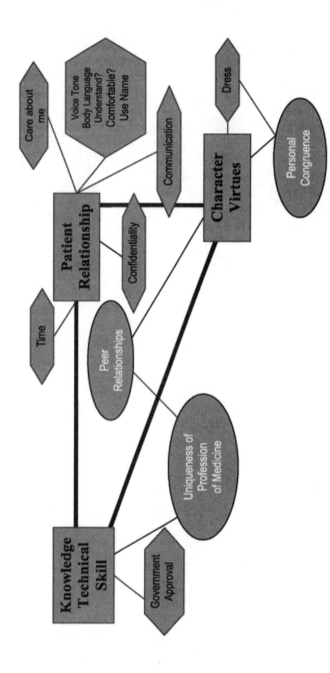

Figure 4.4.   Patient professionalism map.

While all three groups agreed that relationships with patients are important, different aspects of these relationships were emphasized. Highlighted in the article were statements by faculty (attending physicians) about the importance they placed in "patients believ[ing], trust[ing], and hav[ing] total confidence in you," and a balance "between being authoritarian and partnering with patients."

Patients spent the most time emphasizing that they want "caring and compassion, reassurance, and doctors that have time for patients," and physicians who can be "down to earth" and "give hope."

There were also differences in how doctors and patients expressed the importance of good character. While all groups shared certain characteristics in their list, including compassion, only attending physicians listed the characteristic of "maturity." For their part, patients expressed a few aspects of character that were not emphasized by the other groups, including "humor, the ability to show emotion, being down to earth, and honesty."

The authors conclude that the groups do not differ regarding the basic concepts of professionalism but on the relative emphases among them. "The detail of interest" moves among the "concept maps" they display of the three groups. The authors hypothesize that the emphasis shifts from patients (and students, figure not shown here), who focus on relationship, to knowledge and skill, which is more emphasized among attending physicians and junior doctors. Patients care about feeling and communication, while doctors care about seeming reliable and "mature."

In this study, doctors, junior doctors, and patients all agreed on broad categories of professionalism. The difference between "maturity" and "relationship" is an accurate reflection of a dynamic that exists in every patient-doctor encounter. The doctors see themselves as professionals, and patients see themselves—as themselves, wanting to get better, and be cared for by a fellow human being. Yes, this fellow human being should know something (competence is necessary), but he or she should be together with us in a relationship.

THE DOCTOR'S ROLE: BRIDGING THE GAP BETWEEN DOCTORS' VIEWS AND OURS

How can this gap between us and our doctors be bridged? Strategies have been proposed from the point of the view of doctors' associations and societies. One promising idea[10] involves training humanism "connoisseurs," people who can appreciate the humanistic side of medicine and make sure that some aspects of it are reflected in the work of every doctor.

This is great for those who have control over medical education, the training of junior doctors, or the continuing education of attending physicians. As patients, of course, we have none of this. How do we have some input into how doctors see themselves? More important, should we have such input? After all, we are not asked for our advice on professionalism standards for lawyers, plumbers, or clergy, are we?

Maybe such professions should ask for our advice, though. And doctors should most of all. Though the conclusions we can draw from the single study of Wagner et al., are limited, it shows us something important: that doctors, even today, when the pendulum of medical practice has swung back somewhat toward the patient, are still concerned for their professional image. They don't want to come off as suckers. They have a reputation to maintain—they want to appear mature.

How do we insert ourselves into that self-conception of doctors? I don't have any foolproof plan that is supported by the scientific literature, because this is an area that literature hasn't touched yet. I believe, however, that we should make use of suggestion. This suggestion should be open, not subliminal, but it should be subtle. We need to remind and reassure doctors that we respect and care about their professionalism.

How should we do that? It seems strange, the idea that we should reassure our doctors. We are the ones with health problems. Our doctors should be reassuring us! But it's not about doctors' self-esteem. We are not propping them up against their lack of self-confidence—if that were the case, no one would want to be these doctors' patients.

We are acknowledging a doctor's part in the relationship. If we want him or her to recognize our very real concerns and need for our preferences to be expressed, we have to see that the doctor's concerns and preferences are met as well.

ACKNOWLEDGING DOCTORS' PROFESSIONAL NEEDS

Here are some options for such a conversation. Imagine that you have diabetes, and the doctor would like to start you on a medication to treat diabetes by lowering blood sugar. Like many other people, you are pretty sure that you would like to stay away from medicines, especially with all the side effects that you have read about. Given your opposing viewpoints, such a conversation might go like this:

Doctor: Let's talk about your diabetes treatment. I think you need to be on some medication.

Patient: Um....

Doctor: There's a medicine I would like to start you on called metformin. We'll start at 500 milligrams twice a day.

Patient: Do you think this is really necessary?

Doctor: It's really the best choice.

Here no one has really had a conversation about what they want. The doctor has said only, "I would like to start you" on this medication, without really saying why, and the patient has only incompletely expressed her reservations, with the question "Do you think this is really necessary?" Another way to have this conversation, while acknowledging the doctor's need to demonstrate professionalism, might go like this:

Doctor: We need to talk about your diabetes treatment.

Patient: What do you think we should do? What is your expert opinion?

Doctor: Usually, I start people on a medication called metformin. It's a medication to make your body more sensitive to insulin.

Patient: What are other alternatives that you approve of?

Doctor: Well, in certain cases, diabetes can be controlled with close attention to diet and exercise.

Patient: What do you think about those alternatives?

Doctor: To be honest, they don't work in all cases.

Patient: Do you think they're worth a try in a committed patient?

Doctor: I think they might be worth a try, yes.

I know that many doctors are not open to this kind of conversation or such a discussion about treatment. How to change the relationship between you and the doctor in more fundamental ways will be the subject of future chapters. However, to even explore the possibility of forging a relationship-based partnership, respect must be given and granted by both parties. Many doctors do not respect us, and we will talk about that as well—this is both an individual and a systemic problem. But, as we learned from the study by Wagner, et al., doctors see themselves as professionals who are mature and in whom we have confidence, trust, and belief. Think about all the situations in life where we need to interact with authority in a cooperative way without kowtowing or losing our independent opinions. We teach our kids that they have to work together with their teachers even if they don't necessarily agree with them all the time. It's the same way with doctors.

There are a number of similar phrases that might be helpful. We might ask a doctor, "What are some other alternatives that you are familiar with, that your colleagues might use more often than you?" Or, "Are there options that you find popular with your patients?" Another possibility is, "Are there alternative therapies that you think might be worth trying?"

These are not to inculcate blind respect on our part. There is certainly no shortage of tone-deaf, steamrolling, heedless, and even venal doctors. But, as with other professionals, we do not assume that the majority of doctors are like that. The doctor should give us the benefit of the doubt as patients. To do otherwise is the "moral fallacy": that we can blame the obese person for their weight, the drug addict for their drug use, the person with depression for their mental illness. Yes, there is some component of personal responsibility, but our treatment is not based on that alone.

Similarly, the doctor can be blamed for not hearing our complaints, not eliciting our preferences, and generally assuming that health care revolves around them to the exclusion of us. But this blame is only partial, because the doctor has been trained in a system that encourages this. If we want to make possible a workable relationship between them and us, we have to try and take matters into our own hands. We can say things like, "What do you think, in your expert [or professional] opinion?" "As my doctor, what do you think?"

These are not empty phrases. If you have ever brought in scientific literature to your doctor's office to discuss it with him or her, you might have been met by an astonished reaction, or perhaps even an offended grimace. Sure, this wasn't the right reaction for your doctor to show to you, and you have every right to bring supplemental materials into the office. But to build the relationship the materials need to be presented in the proper context.

PATIENTS SHOULD BE INVOLVED IN DEFINING THE DOCTOR'S ROLE

There's a larger issue here. The concept of professionalism that we have discussed up to now is insufficient. It involves only the doctor's self-definition, or to be generous, the self-definition of doctors that large groups of them have worked out for themselves.

The process of arriving at these definitions involves glaring deficiencies. What do we patients think about how doctors define themselves? Is there a way these patient opinions can be incorporated into current definitions of professionalism? As I have mentioned, medical education is now ever more concerned with training doctors to be listening people as well as technical experts. What happens after training is customarily limited to the realm of "continuing medical education," courses that doctors take to maintain their licensure and certification.

One way to make sure that both patients and doctors pay attention to a bilateral relationship is for doctors to mention their relationship with patients in their definitions of professionalism. But not only that—these definitions should also mention what the needs of the doctor are in this relationship, so that the relationship can be conducted on a basis of mutual respect.

The other glaring deficiency in current definitions of professionalism, as is pointed out by the Wagner study, is the lack of a statement of how the doctor is meant to connect to the society at large. This matters to a patient's relationship with the doctor, even though doctors might not see it that way. [11]

Many people don't think much about public health and how it connects to their own individual health. Later in this book we will discuss the connection between healthy relationships and healthy populations. First, though, we must help doctors modify their self-conception, their definition of professionalism, to encompass the health of populations.

Why? Because doctors are imperfect just like we are all imperfect. We all are motivated by transient biases and fleeting stereotypes; we have learned above that doctors are susceptible to these biases too—not because they are bad people but because they are just like everyone else. What do we do about these biases? We can try and teach empathy. [12] Training programs can try to teach doctors to recognize racism, for example through educational videos, [13] though I don't know of any good scientific evidence that such videos work, much less that teaching doctors to recognize racism actually reduces its prevalence in the examination room.

A more scientifically based way to combat such biases, and one more likely to appeal to doctors' necessary self-image of respect and maturity, is to connect public health to patient health. Like anyone else, doctors use stereotypes because they mistakenly think that specific cases can be indiscriminately applied to general situations. Sometimes that is the case—there are medications for high blood pressure that work better in African Americans than in other populations—but not all the time. The only way to connect groups of people to the individual person in a scientifically reliable way so that the individual is helped, is through public health. If we approach doctors with this change to their definition of professionalism (that they should consider the health of populations, not just individuals), they might complain. It is enough for them, they would say, to take care of one person at a time. How can they be expected to treat the whole world?

Imagine that you go to a doctor to treat your diabetes. She wants to discuss your diet with you, and asks you what kind if carbohydrates you eat and uses the example of bread or noodles. You are from a cultural group that eats rice, and you don't think this example is relevant—for, after all, rice is a nourishing food and necessary for health! Everyone knows that! Only if the doctor understands the connection between culture and person can she, in your case, help you understand what elements of your diet need to be changed. You can call this cultural competence or diversity if you like, but it's really public health.

We started this chapter talking about the first, or at least most famous, statement of medical professionalism: the Hippocratic Oath. The most widely cited scholarly work on the Oath, by the classical scholar Ludwig Edelstein, says with finality that "the Hippocratic Oath is a Pythagorean manifesto and not the expression of an absolute standard of medical conduct."[14] But every statement of professionalism can be read as a manifesto of the time in which it is written. Our present time is one of huge technological advance and cost, with parallel realization that much of this technology does not contribute to health or well-being. It is an age of fragmented health care, where people may see a number of different doctors during their lifetime. It is an age when the connection between population health and individual health continues to be realized, if only passively. And, finally, we know now that the relationship between doctor and patient can be nearly as important as any single medication, procedure, or test.

Given all these facts, we need a statement of the ideals that doctors aspire to—their professionalism—which is in keeping with them. That will help prepare doctors to have a healing relationship with their patients, at the same time as patients give them the respect and standing they need. The next time a group of doctors meets to consider their vision of their profession, they should include the opinions of us patients and widen their vision to include not just their relationship to us as individuals, but to the health of society at large.

Chapter Five

Measuring How Good Our Doctors Are

In every hospital and clinic across the country, doctors are talking about quality. There are two impulses behind this conversation. One is that the federal government has begun to pay doctors more if they demonstrate greater quality, and deny them that extra money if they don't. The other is the widespread assumption that patients will begin to choose those hospitals and doctors that demonstrate greater quality.

The first statement is a bald fact. We'll talk about what incentives the government now has in place to encourage quality, and which of them are justified. But the second assumption is more complicated. I don't know who chooses their doctor because they are of higher "quality."

WHAT IS QUALITY?

As with so many things, we have to start with definitions. What does quality mean? There are two ways to approach it. One is through particular processes. Doctors pursue quality when they complete those actions, tests, or treatments that are the best, which are supported by the best available evidence. Higher quality in diabetes, for example, means checking the hemoglobin A1C blood test every three months, which shows how high the blood sugar has been; performing an eye exam and checking the feet every year; and achieving goals for blood pressure and cholesterol. Whole industries and branches of government have sprung up in recent decades encouraging doctors and hospitals to aim for these goals.

What "quality" means for the doctor or hospital, no matter what disease we're talking about, could be as simple as adding together the list of "what should be done" for every disease. So, for example, we would take the list of "what every doctor should do" for diabetes, heart disease, pneumonia, and obesity, and voila, we would have the definition of a quality doctor or hospital for anyone suffering from one of those diseases.

In the first part of this chapter, I will talk about how we can make such a definition of quality work—because it makes a lot of sense and it's worthwhile following in many instances. In the second part of this chapter, I will talk about how this definition can be very misleading, and distort what both we and our doctors are trying to do.

QUALITY BY CHECKLIST

The definition of quality that involves counting up what doctors should be doing can be called the "checklist" method. Checklists have been made famous by a number of doctors lately, including Atul Gawande[1] and Peter Pronovost.[2] In the writings of these authors, the term is generally used to refer to situations in which there is an easily defined sequence of events that leads to a better outcome. For example, if someone needs to have a catheter inserted into a vein or artery in the intensive care unit, it can be done with very little risk of bloodstream infection. Pronovost's checklist lists the steps that doctors should take to prevent this in every situation. Gawande takes this principle and expands it to other areas of health care.

Both Pronovost and Gawande come from medical specialties where the need is often acute: Pronovost is an anesthesiologist who trained in intensive care units, and Gawande is a general surgeon. Of course, they are thoughtful and deliberate, and both have devoted much of their work to a careful working out of what should be in checklists and how to disseminate them once that content has been decided.

But most of our time in the health care system is not spent in an intensive-care bed or an operating room—it's spent in a "regular" bed in a hospital or face-to-face with a health care provider in a clinic. How does the notion of checklist apply to these situations?

PROCESS OR OUTCOME—WHICH IS MORE IMPORTANT?

"Checklist" is shorthand, but we should focus on a careful definition of quality. Health researchers and doctors have always quarreled about the relative importance of process versus outcomes.

Outcomes include whether we die or are sick. Process refers to things that happen along the way. Outcomes for diabetes, for example, include whether our blood sugar levels (often measured by the hemoglobin A1C) are in control, whether our blood pressure is in the right place, or whether our cholesterol is in a certain range. These "process measures" are only as good as the evidence connecting them to outcomes, but sometimes these measures are all we have. Indeed, sometimes it takes years for new process measures to be proposed, vetted, and found useful. The best predictors of future heart disease are still the tried and true variety: blood pressure, cholesterol, smoking, diabetes, and a family history of early heart disease. While new tests have been proposed as an addition to this list, none of them have yet been found to provide information that's better than these basic predictors.

Sometimes we have the outcome available to measure—someone contracts a bloodstream infection from an implanted catheter—and sometimes we only have process measures. The process measures are likely to be our proxies for the outcomes when we are preventing events that are hard to measure over the short or medium term. For instance, when doctors treat us for high blood pressure or diabetes, it makes no sense to declare success if we are alive without a new heart attack or stroke at the end of, say, six months. That's why process measures are used as a proxy.

To use process measures in this way is not as simple as all that, of course. Complications ensue at every stage of the process. First, it isn't always clear what the best outcomes to measure would be. Obviously, if we had heart disease, and the alternative to dying sooner with a heart attack were easily tolerable medications, we could quickly make our peace with such inconvenience for the sake of longer life.

But for other diseases, it's not so easy. For example, more and more people are found to have breast cancer, because mammograms are widely recommended. Mammograms find cancer earlier, but it doesn't mean people live longer because of their mammograms—rather, it means that the clock has been started earlier (owing to the earlier diagnosis of cancer), with more time artificially tacked on to the survival clock. It's like those people who call themselves thirty-nine years old for a year and a half: it doesn't make them any younger, it just moves the goalposts back.

Most difficult are those diseases without so-called hard endpoints. Even if diabetes is not by itself a cause of death, there are increased rates of other complications that are associated with diabetes—for example, heart attacks, strokes, and infections. But what about someone who has chronic pain and goes to a doctor? The doctor is often not going to be able to make the pain go away, so comparing one doctor to another on this basis would be over-optimistic, even unfair. How are we going to tell if the doctor is providing "quality" care to us if we have that pain? Should we decide beforehand on a measure of improvement in the pain that the doctor should achieve? Fifty percent? A level of 3 or below on a 1 to 10 scale? What if it's just implausible that the pain would be improved to such an extent?

Another area where the most important outcomes are not always obvious is the care of patients with cancer. Not all cancers are the same. Some can be cured and many more cannot. There are a number of different tumors for which chemotherapy is available. Chemotherapy can extend survival, but at the price of intolerable side effects. And survival might not be extended for more than a few months. If you had a diagnosis of cancer, which doctor would you say had the highest quality: the one who provided the therapy that minimized side effects, the one who tried to provide the greatest survival, or the doctor who was most assiduous about taking your preferences into account?

Not every disease naturally presents us with endpoints that are easy to interpret, in other words. And not every disease provides surrogates, process measures that mean the same thing to everyone. Does quality mean a lower blood pressure or the lowest, safest blood pressure? Or, even more defined, the lowest, safest blood pressure that is most tolerated by the person taking the medications? Which do we choose when rating the quality of a doctor?

HOW DO WE PATIENTS DEFINE QUALITY?

The lack of a universal, widely agreed-upon definition of quality is one reason behind the recent popularity of patient-reported outcomes.[3] Why not ask us patients to identify the most important results of our care? We could do this in multiple ways. One way would be to ask us our opinion about the disease we have, and what it would take for us to say, "It improved, the doctor did it, and this is what we mean by quality."

If we have diabetes, what do we consider most important about our treatment for the disease? Do we want the rates of big, important outcomes (things that might kill us) to be decreased in the doctor or hospital that we might eventually choose, when comparing them to other doctors or hospitals? Do we want to decrease the number of medications we are on, minimize the out-of-pocket costs that we need to pay, or make sure we are exposed to only a very rare chance of side effects? Or do we want to make sure that we feel as good as possible while we are being treated?

Thus, there can be great diversity in the outcomes, or even in the process measures, that are associated with particular health conditions. But we would like to rate the quality of doctors, or hospitals, across all their patients. (We would like to compare them for various specific diseases, too, but that should be a simpler matter.) Thus, we should agree on a list of aspects that all of us, no matter what our health issues, find important when we go to a doctor or hospital, and find essential to how we think of their quality.

Let's see if we can agree on such a list. We all want to be treated with respect when we go to a doctor; we want the doctor to listen to us and treat us like a human being. We want an emotional connection. Further, we want the doctor to demonstrate a level of technical competence.

In addition, we don't want to be made to wait for our appointment. If we are in the hospital, we don't want to be one of those patients who never seems to meet the attending physician. We also want the medical team as a whole to have the same characteristics as the doctor.

There are further criteria we want to be met. We want our health care to be provided in a safe way. Indeed, quality as a movement grows out of the increasing attention to safety. We want the risk of infection to be kept as low as possible. If any procedures are done, or medications given, they should be done and given for the right person (us!), for the right part of our body, and at the right time.

At this point, we can divide the criteria we have discussed into three categories:

- Safety criteria (what we don't want to happen)
- Process and outcome measures (what we want to happen)
- What we think is important (what people call "patient-related outcomes")

Perhaps we can make headway now. We just need to agree on a minimum set of standards in all three of these categories, apply them across all doctors and all hospitals, and then pick the best doctor or hospital.

WHICH DOCTORS AND HOSPITALS ARE THE BEST, AND HOW DO WE DECIDE?

In fact, the strategy in the previous paragraph is being adopted with lightning speed as you read this book, or at least with as much speed as an entrenched health care and political bureaucracy can muster. *Consumer Reports*, the publication associated with the consumer-advocacy organization Consumers Union, recently posted ratings of hospitals on its website for the first time.[4] This is a big step forward. While the federal government (in the form of the Center for Medicare and Medicaid Services Hospital Compare site) has long made this information available,[5] there isn't much in the scientific literature yet about whether "ordinary people" (i.e., us patients) are using the site. I very much doubt it, because in a survey of primary care doctors done in 2012,[6] only 16 percent were even aware of the site, and "none used publicly reported quality data in referral decisions." The theory behind such quality information is that we will use it to make decisions about doctors and hospitals, and thus doctors and hospitals will need to improve their quality. Perhaps a widely known site like Consumer Reports can bring this information to more people's attention.

Until that day, however, it's a different kind of quality information that is most used by ordinary people. My workplace, Johns Hopkins Hospital, has been named "Best Hospital in America" twenty-one years running in the rankings of *U.S. News*.[7] Of course, I'm not complaining—it makes my employer look good and doesn't hurt me any. The ratings are quite popular, as evidenced by the fact that highly ranked institutions widely publicize the information. The *U.S. News* issue with the rankings does well enough that it's still published in a paper version, though the rest of the magazine has converted to an online-only format.

The *U.S. News* rankings are meant to "to help people who find themselves in need of unusually skilled inpatient care." That is, they are meant to help patients choose hospitals which might provide them the most specialized of procedures: not joint replacements, cataract surgeries, and hernia repairs, which are done at many institutions, but cardiac bypass surgeries or minimally invasive robotic procedures, which are more rareified.

There are several components to the *U.S. News* rankings as they were implemented in 2012 and before.[8] Thirty-two and a half percent comes from reputation; thirty-two and a half percent comes from a "survival score", thirty percent comes from "other care factors," and only five percent comes from hospital-reported data that has to do with safety. (For several specialties, not enough information is available for the domains besides reputation, so that is the only one used to make the score.)

It is curious that only five percent comes from safety data—but maybe we don't actually care about such information when choosing hospitals. More interesting is whether or not the *U.S. News* rankings actually give us additional, useful information we can use when choosing a hospital. Ashwini Sehgal, a cardiologist at Case Western Reserve University in Cleveland, published an interesting analysis in 2010 in the top-flight journal *Annals of Internal Medicine*.[9] He found that the specialty's number 1-ranked hospitals could be predicted by reputation alone—100 percent of the time. The ten top ranked hospitals in each specialty could be predicted by reputation alone 91 percent of the time.

U.S. News changed the methodology of the "Best Hospitals Guide" in 2012–2013 to focus marginally less on reputation. There's a larger issue here, however, which makes the business of rating hospitals or doctors questionable: do people actually use these ratings when choosing health care?

WHAT INFORMATION DO WE USE TO CHOOSE HEALTH CARE?

I. B. DeGroot and other researchers in The Netherlands conducted a survey of 337 new surgical patients, asking them for the basis of their hospital choice.[10] While we should keep in mind that the study was done in another country, the results are striking.

Not surprisingly, people who compared hospitals to each other used publicly available information on hospitals more often than those who did not compare hospitals to each other. The surprise is in how little they used such information. Of those who reported comparing hospitals, only 12.7 percent made use of public reporting. (Of those who reported not comparing hospitals, only 1.5 percent did so.) What information did people use in this study? Most relied on their own (48 percent) and other people's experiences (31 percent).

Perhaps we choose hospitals and doctors the way we choose so many other things, through reputation. We ask our friends and family members. Doctors certainly rely on reputation when their patients ask them for referrals. Is such reputation-based hospital choice good or bad—does it lead us to choose better or worse hospitals? A study done twenty-five years ago might give some answer. In an article in the *Journal of the American Medical Association*, Howard Luft, et al., examined whether—in the era before public reporting of hospital information—patients' choice of hospitals depended on hospitals' characteristics. [11]

Luft and the co-authors found that hospitals were less likely to be chosen if they were farther away from the respondent, and more likely if they were affiliated with a medical school. The authors correlated the likelihood of choosing a hospital among a subset of surgical procedures and medical diagnoses. For some of those procedures and diagnoses, but not all, hospitals with poorer than expected outcomes attracted fewer patients.

To summarize: neither we nor our doctors often make use of publicly available information that compares the quality of doctors and hospitals. Even when we do, we care a lot more about the reputation of the doctor or hospital we are thinking about using. There doesn't seem to be much literature about the way doctors use reputation in referring someone to a colleague, but it seems plausible that they use it just as we patients do. A widespread rating system for hospitals that these hospitals go out of their way to publicize, is based not on "quality measures" but on that same criteria—reputation.

THE FLAWS OF QUALITY MEASUREMENT

This points to the weakness of measuring quality in doctors and hospitals, a weakness that can be pictured as three tottering, crumbling pillars.

Pillar 1: We don't know what we *are* measuring—that is, we don't know enough about the quality of our information.

Pillar 2: We don't know what we *should be* measuring.

Pillar 3: We don't know how what we measure connects to what we should be doing to improve our health.

We'll take the pillars one by one.

We don't know what we're measuring: There is good news and bad news. We have information on the characteristics of doctors and hospitals that make intuitive sense to us, which would make us more likely to recommend them to friends. For example, the HCAHPS (Hospital Care Quality Information from the Consumer Perspective) questionnaires[12] include questions on "Communication with Nurses, Communication with Doctors, Responsiveness of Hospital Staff, Pain Management, and Communication about Medicine," as well as questions about "Cleanliness of Hospital Environment and Quietness of Hospital Environment." Sounds great, and certainly these things ring true intuitively as part of quality. They measure what most people consider important to their satisfaction. In fact, the Hospital Compare website includes the HCAHPS survey in its statistics.

However, if you look at the response rates to the HCAHPS surveys sent to people discharged from the hospital from January to December 2010, you start to see a problem.[13] The response rates range from 13 percent in the Virgin Islands to 43 percent in Iowa. I don't know why the response rate is lower in the Virgin Islands. Somewhat more concerning is the absence of Puerto Rico from the list.

More disquieting are the response rates themselves. Imagine if you had to organize a lunch party for your office and you managed to find fewer than half the people at work to ask them what kind of sandwich they liked. Or, even more germane, imagine if you worked at a large company manufacturing airplanes, and you had to survey airlines about possible sources of error or malfunction in your product. However, you spilled coffee over more than half of your address book. This is what the HCAHPS is measuring—data on satisfaction that is only half complete.

Let's be fair, though. A 100 percent response rate is impossible, especially for mailed surveys. The question is whether those who did respond are representative of everyone. They are probably not. The people who fail to send in their answers are not those who had an impeccable experience, but those who don't want to think about it anymore. I am speculating, but it is very plausible that we are systematically overestimating how satisfied people are with their experience in the hospital.

But the problems go even deeper. We don't know what we *should be* measuring. What are those measures of communication that are most closely connected to improved health? We have already talked about a few plausible guesses: doctors should let us fully express our chief complaint, be open to our emotional needs, and let us express our preferences for how the visit should go. We should set the agenda. In future chapters, I'll talk about being mindful to what the doctor is saying, and he or she being mindful, in return, to us—with such reciprocal communication building a healthy relationship. But, though I shouldn't say this in a book that is trying to convince you of the importance of communication, the connection of communication to clinically important outcomes is not yet a rock-solid scientific fact.

The examples of heart disease and diabetes are instructive. We know what is associated with heart disease: high blood pressure, high cholesterol, smoking, diabetes, and a family history of heart disease. Occasionally, new lab tests are suggested that will help predict people's future risk of heart disease if the other factors aren't abnormal enough to make the call.

For diabetes, however, there is an ongoing dispute about just where someone's blood sugar should be to prevent diseases from rearing their heads later in life: conditions such as heart attack, stroke, eye disease, kidney failure, or disease of the blood vessels resulting in amputated limbs. The blood test used is the Hemoglobin A1C, which measures the amount of sugar attached to blood cells in the form of glycoprotein. Since these blood cells hang around in the bloodstream, the test is representative of the blood sugar levels over the past three months. There has been a back and forth over the past few years about what number we should target with this blood test.[14] With time, doctors have become wiser, or at least more knowledgeable, about the trade-off between aggressive treatment of diabetes (making the blood sugar, and thus the hemoglobin A1C, lower) and the side effects that accompany any treatment.

In regard to the factors that are connected to hospital and doctor quality (Pillar 2), we are not as well placed as we are with heart disease, for which many of the relevant factors (what we should be measuring) are already known. On the other hand, the factors related to quality are not as controversial as is the "perfect" value of the hemoglobin A1C in diabetes. We know about certain things that are associated with quality, especially those outcomes that are connected to patient safety: rates of blood stream infections from catheter insertions; frequency of hand washing; how often surgery is done at the wrong site; whether infections with multiple drug-resistant staphylococcus aureus are screened for at the hospital; the frequency of medication errors. My colleague Peter Pronovost at Johns Hopkins has helped make the world aware of these problems.[15]

But, apart from the bigger fish of safety issues, what about all the "other" stuff that happens in the hospital, the stuff that the HCAHPS surveys address? What about communication between us and our doctors making sure we are on the same page, that our concerns are addressed, questions answered, and preferences heard and taken into account? What about making sure that all the doctors in the hospital talk to each other? What about taking steps to check that the institution—be it hospital or clinic—is acting the way we would want any institution that interacts with us to operate: with respect, responsibility, and decent human values?

This "other" category is only partially measured. Which of the factors above should we measure? How do we best do it? And how do we connect Pillars 2 and 3? That is to say, we could very well embark on a nationwide mission to identify and promote the most important elements of doctor-patient communication in the hospital. We could agree on standards and definitions; create nationwide databases on what doctors, nurses, and hospitals do right or wrong. A national institute could get behind these results and issue recommendations. In short, we could do for communication what Peter Pronovost and his colleagues have done for hospital safety. We could do the same thing for what people dismissively call the "soft endpoints" of medical care: patient satisfaction, for instance, could be treated the same way.

But Pillar 3 requires that we know the connection between these findings and better health. If doctors communicate better in the hospital, will we live longer or have fewer heart attacks? For most endpoints, we have no idea. For some, obviously, we do: there is some evidence that better communication can lead to greater adherence to doctors' recommendations for the treatment of pain, which—in turn—leads to improved pain control.[16] But the connection between communication and outcomes is not yet obvious across the board.

This doesn't mean that communication should not be pursued—obviously it should, for reasons of ethics and esthetics: it's the right thing to do and it feels right. Also, I have no doubt that communication will indeed be associated with a broad array of positive health outcomes, as is now known to be the case for a narrower range.

WILL REGULATIONS ENSURE QUALITY?

What we can't do is assume that legislating communication improvement in the name of quality will automatically ensure better health. This is the cardinal mistake of the quality movement. Trying to modify the behavior of doctors through incentives or regulation can lead them in the opposite direction entirely.

Imagine that you come to see a doctor, and she tells you that you need a mammogram—it's the recommended thing to do. You discuss the risks and benefits with her, and you decide that, no, in fact, you would rather not have the mammogram. The doctor pushes you a little bit, but you stand your ground. The mammograms are painful, you've had them many times in the past, and if you're going to get cancer—you might think—you're going to get cancer.

From the doctor's point of view, there will be ever more pressure to deliver the goods with regard to quality metrics. Today there are regulations that peg the reimbursement that a clinic or practice receives to the meeting of certain targets, if that clinic or practice is based at a hospital. One of these might be mammography: a practice might be rewarded, or not penalized, if their mammography rate reaches 90 percent, for example. [17]

Thus the clinic or hospital has a powerful incentive to increase its mammography rates as much as possible. There is a danger that people who do not agree to the favored test might be depreciated, ignored, or pressured. More likely—and more worrisome, perhaps—is that we might do what we do in so many other situations when we see a doctor: keep our objections to ourselves and not say what we're really thinking, out of fear that we will disturb the balance and not be thought of as a good patient. More to the point, mammogram targets will be achieved without waiting for strong and satisfying evidence that the risk-benefit balance makes their universal promotion worthwhile.

I am not against mammograms. But, like any procedure, they have risk and are not wholly benign. The problem is that the big guns of insurance incentives—on the state and the federal level—are being quickly trundled into place, aimed squarely at both doctor and patient. The three-pillar problem, like the issue with quality data for doctors and hospitals, applies to all tests or treatments.

Pillar 1. Do we have reliable information that the tests and treatments encouraged by the rush to "quality" (e.g., HEDIS [Healthcare Effectiveness Data and Information Set]) actually measure what they are supposed to? When your doctor checks your blood pressure, is it a reliable measure? No. [18] Usually it's not taken according to the recommendations of people who have thought about the issue the most, and this affects how doctors recommend blood-pressure treatment.

Pillar 2. Are we sure that the "quality metrics" that institutions are rapidly adopting are the ones we should be measuring? Should doctors be given incentives to make sure that the hemoglobin A1C (the measure of diabetes control we discussed above) is under 7, 8, or 9 percent? Which is most important: that people with diabetes have an eye exam, smokers be helped to quit, or patients suffering from depression be directed to treatment?

Choosing among those alternatives is difficult, because we don't have studies to tell us which incentives should be aimed at which problems in what order. Even more difficult (and this is Pillar 3) is that we don't know what health benefit to expect from racing after the quality, even if we had well-founded measurements (Pillar 1) of the right objectives (Pillar 2). What if we measured hypertension, encouraged doctors to treat it, and found out after all that we weren't making people healthier?

But why would that be? Why would pushing doctors to do the right thing not make people healthier or live longer? There are a number of possible reasons—not everyone takes their medicine; not every medicine works; some people have heart problems and get sick from them even if their blood pressure is controlled—but underlying these reasons is one principle:

Evidence can keep doctors from making the wrong decision, but it can never ensure they are making the right decision for an individual.

Whenever you talk to your doctor about a medical decision, and he or she uses words like "must" or "should," "recommendation" or "guideline," you should wonder on what basis the evidence or guideline is supported, and what the alternatives are. The problem with quality is not that there's something wrong with encouraging doctors to do the right thing rather than the wrong thing. Doctors do many wrong things, such as ordering procedures because they are fashionable or because they will get reimbursed for them, rather than for any scientifically sound reason.[19]

But doctors also need encouragement to do the right thing in a way that is specific to us, the patients. We need to take our time with such quality initiatives, ensuring that what we are incentivizing doctors to do are the right things, in the right way, at the right time, supported by the best evidence.

The job of finding the best evidence, figuring out the most important tests, and establishing the connections between those tests and our health—pillars 1, 2, and 3—are not the patients' job. That's the job of doctors and scientists. What patients have to be is the bridge from science and the doctor's recommendations (often imperfect and falsely presented as incontrovertible) to our own interests and preferences. To do that we have to learn how to express our preferences in the context of the visit with our doctor—which starts even before our appointment. That is the topic of the next chapter.

Chapter Six

Telling Our Story: Taking the Time to Express Our Health Concerns to Ourselves and Others

Nearly all of us will see a doctor at some point: over 80 percent of Americans saw a health care professional sometime in the past year.[1] Early on, it's important we learn how to talk to doctors so that we are heard and our concerns addressed. Perhaps a good way to go about it is to learn how to express our health problems and concerns clearly and understandably in a way that points to the underlying issues. This may take practice; it might require notes or even a partner to come along. When we walk into a doctor's office for the first time, we could do so confidently, with the knowledge that we have practiced how to do these things beforehand.

Of course, things are never this simple. Many health care encounters occur in urgent circumstances, when we are panicked, confused, and scared. And even when a matter is not urgent, before we pick a primary care doctor (our regular doctor) and make an appointment to see her in the office, there are plenty of people we usually talk to. We might ask for advice from a friend, partner, or family member; often we consult online sources. We hem and haw about whether an issue requires medical attention, deciding whether or not this is the right thing to see the doctor about. We might even button-hole a doctor or nurse whom we know personally, who is not "our" doctor, just because our preexisting relationship with him outside of a doctor's office makes it realistic to approach him and ask questions without feeling uncomfortable.

When we finally make the decision to see a doctor, we can't just waltz in and see one, or at least, not how the current system is designed. We need to present our symptoms and our reason for seeing the doctor several times before we step over the threshold. Each one of these times is an opportunity for us to frame our thoughts, clarify to ourselves which symptoms we think are important and why, and prepare ourselves for a visit that might not be as definitive or as long as we like.

COMMUNICATING EVEN BEFORE THE VISIT

This area of "pre-visit communication" is under-researched because it spans a variety of different domains. In the privacy of our home, we realize something might be wrong with our body. Perhaps something hurts, or we are short of breath. Or we have a problem with our medication. Or it might be something even more serious. We feel as though our world is upended and we have nothing to live for. It could even be an unclear feeling that we don't feel safe or healthy. Our first responsibility is to pay attention to our own body and understand whether a symptom is important or not. The relevant term in the social sciences is "framing," that is, everything has a context. We don't interpret facts in a vacuum: what might be a tic to one person might seem like a wink to another. Similarly, we should be able to tell a story about the symptom that is bothering us, at the very least to ourselves. We should be able to convey a coherent narrative about our symptoms.[2] Our symptoms belong to us uniquely, but it is our job to tell the doctors a story about them. This is not going to be the same story they would tell in medical language, but a clear account of when the symptoms started, what part of our body they affected, what made them better or worse, what treatment we have pursued up to now, and whether they have happened before. We should include aspects of the symptoms that many people feel uncomfortable sharing with their doctor: what we are worried about, and what these symptoms make us think of.

In practicing a narrative—preparing a story for the person you will see in the office—you are not playacting or "telling a story" in the sense of perpetrating a falsehood. It's a matter of framing. Remind yourself of situations when you prepared before talking to someone, whether asking someone for a date, requesting a raise from your boss, going on a job interview, or giving a report at school. All of these required preparation, so why shouldn't a visit to the doctor require the same thing? When it comes to our health, telling the story of how we got here may be just as important as recording the symptoms in real time.

But this is not just any preparation. It's not just about writing up a convincing speech. You are not putting your case to a lawyer, after all, but trying to build a partnership with your doctor. You want them to understand your situation but not think you are groveling or a wimp. Many of us care what our doctor thinks of us, even if only implicitly. That's why when we tell the doctor about our pains or other symptoms, we often make sure we call them "minor" or "just a little thing," so as not to seem difficult or complaining. This can be misleading. We want to tell the truth. We should be able to tell the doctor how our symptoms truly make us feel.

In other words, you want to put not your best, but your most authentic, foot forward, the story that most accurately portrays how your symptom or disease makes you feel. Two examples will illustrate what I mean. These are taken from people that saw me as a doctor, though they are of course modified to eliminate any information that could identify them.

Patient 1: A. R.: 68-year-old man

> I took my nitroglycerin pills regularly over the last few months because of my blood pressure. I don't know what's going on, but I think my blood pressure must be up, because I know that's a problem I have. I don't think it's a problem, it's probably just a little thing. Would you check my blood pressure just to make sure it's not up again?

Patient 2: Y. A.: 45-year-old woman

> Something's wrong, I have a pain here [points to her left side] and here [points to her right side]. I don't remember when it started, and I'm not sure what makes it better or worse. I know my kidneys are located here [points to her back], so maybe it has something to do with that?

Patients 1 and 2 are cognitively normal and interact more or less as anyone their age would with people in daily life. The way they present their symptoms, however, doesn't reflect how they feel them; we can tell this through how they frame their symptoms. "I know that my blood pressure is up," for example, is a legitimate interpretation on the part of Patient 1, but it is not what he is feeling. There might be people who feel something in their body and say, "Hey, that's my blood pressure," for example, without first thinking about their immediate physical symptom, but I don't know them.

Patient 2 doesn't remember much about her pain. That's understandable, especially if you feel bad in an episodic way; you might not remember to write down how or what you're feeling and when you're feeling bad, before the feeling itself passes and you're left with only the conviction that you should see the doctor about something that doesn't feel quite right.

But it's also likely that Patient 2 just didn't realize that noting such things might be useful to communicating with the doctor. Recording these details might also be useful in communicating with the number of people we might have to interact with before we see the doctor. Usually, our visit with our provider happens only after we pass through several layers that feel like hoops to jump through. There's the person on the phone making our appointment, then the medical assistant or nurse, then the doctor. The doctor himself might not even be "our doctor," but the partner in the group practice who is available to see us on that particular day. It takes repetition to convey messages. The earlier we get started framing our own message to ourselves, and practicing that framing, the more accurately we can tell each member of the health-care team what we are feeling and what we think needs to be done to make it better.

HOW TO TELL ABOUT OUR SYMPTOMS: SOME PRACTICAL STEPS

The first step is to *take an active role in recording our symptoms*. This serves several purposes. First, it's a record of the ups and downs of our problems. Second, it's an admission and an affirmation to ourselves that we take these symptoms seriously. Paradoxically, taking our problems seriously like this might make it more difficult to start recording. If we start writing down our symptoms, it means they are not going away anytime soon and we have to deal with them. That's why putting pen to paper, or finger to keyboard, is necessary—to get over that feeling.

And such a symptom diary can actually be therapeutic in itself. Much as spiritual masters have used diaries to keep track of their own moral development, we can use the diary to advance our understanding of our physical selves. Last, of course, this symptom diary gives our doctor or nurse something to go on, a context in which to place and examine the symptom or group of symptoms. Even a sheet as simple as this can be helpful:

Date:_____
Pain (Yes/No)
Sleep Last Night (Good/Bad)
Alcohol Last Night (Yes/No)

The sheet can be made more detailed, with pain ratings, maps of your body to depict where your symptoms are, and times of day. The point is not necessarily to present your doctor with this record of your body's changes—though that can be very useful in certain cases—but to make it easier for you to understand your own story.

The second step is to *be honest about what you think is going on*. You know your own body and are the world's foremost expert on how you perceive your symptoms. Saying "I'm not sure what I have" or "I actually don't know what this is" is not a harmless hedge but a potential disavowal of seriousness that works against your own interests.

Even if you are saying it as a gesture of respect to the doctor, so as not to be thought a complainer, it could be dangerous if you are withholding potentially useful information. If you just learned that your friend or relative was diagnosed with cancer and you are worried sick for that reason about your lump or bump, say that. If you have had tightness in your chest for the past few months, you can put that information in context without seeming like a whiner or a wimp. If you don't have the terrible disease you are worried about, wouldn't you prefer the doctor to reassure you that it is, in fact, something else?

The third step is to *be explicit about what you are looking for from your visit* with the doctor and use that to help you tell your story. If you are sure that a certain sort of medication will help your pain, say that. If you—as in the example above—are terrified that your lump signifies cancer, make that the conclusion of your tale.

Obviously, if you truly don't know what is going on, haven't managed to keep track of your symptoms, and don't know what you want from the doctor, then there is no way you can truthfully massage your needs and experiences into a narrative, and the suggestions above might not apply to you. There are other ways you can organize the visit to build a relationship.

But here are some examples of narratives that work to show you what I am talking about:

Patient 3. F. S.: 35 year-old woman.

> I've had some eye problems over the years, I have been to doctors and most of them just think I have dry eyes. I have been given some drops and my symptoms have gone away. But a week ago my eye started to tear and sting. I am worried it's an infection because there's yellow . . . stuff coming out of it. I'm pretty sure I need an antibiotic and that's why I'm making an appointment for today.

This woman has thought about the things that are bothering her and built a narrative around them. She has started out with her history, continued with what is bothering her currently, talked about her worries, and mentioned what she needs and expects from her appointment. Here's another example for a problem that is not simple and a lot of people experience.

Patient 4. T. L.: 58-year-old man.

> I've had pain for a long time and I don't know if it's ever going away. I hurt all over. I've seen what feels like a hundred doctors, they've done a bunch of tests, and everyone says they don't know what's causing my pain. I wish there were something someone could do to make it go away. I am taking some medications for my pain but they don't work. Is there anything stronger that

won't make me sick? Also, are there any tests we can do to figure out the source of my pain? No one has listened to me before, so I hope you can help me.

This narrative is different from the previous one, because the person recounting it is clearly desperate. Anyone hearing it is likely not going to be put at their ease. This pain is most likely also not going to get better, as is the case with most chronic pain sufferers. Still, this narrative is presented in a way that represents the needs and ideas of the person suffering the pain.

Once you have constructed such a narrative, what do you do with it? It's not something you memorize, like a part in a school play, but something you internalize to better understand how you might present your symptoms to someone who asks about them. You should make several versions of this narrative. When we call the secretary or office coordinator to try and make an appointment with our doctor, we need to catch her attention and help her to understand the importance of our condition without being annoying. We might have just a few minutes over the phone. This might be something as short as, "I'm having a lot of pain and I need to ask the doctor about it," or "I want to ask the doctor about my medicines."

Phoning your doctor's office involves a little bit more than just presenting the narrative of your symptoms. When you call a doctor's office to make an appointment or speak with someone, there is usually a message when you are put on hold. "If this is a life-threatening emergency," the message might say, "please call 911."

How do you know if it is a life-threatening emergency? Obviously, if you have any suspicion at all that what you feel is life-threatening, you should probably err on the side of going to the emergency room. I am not going to be the one to de-emphasize your potentially dangerous symptoms.

But there is a big gray area between life-threatening symptoms and everyday aches and pains. If a new symptom comes up, how do we know what sort it is? How much attention should we pay to it? Obviously, there are urgent and serious symptoms that should make us go to the emergency room—for example, any of the widely publicized warning signs of stroke or heart attack. On the other hand, there is always going to be a gray area of symptoms that we are not sure about—should we call 911 or the doctor? Thus this is yet another situation where the way we present our symptoms and concerns can make all the difference in how we are received by the person on the other end of the telephone.

Once we make the appointment, we might be meeting a nurse or medical assistant. More and more often these days, and especially with the widespread adoption of various electronic medical records, we meet at least one person, who enters preliminary information into the medical record template, including the reason you are coming to see the doctor, before you see that doctor. This is where the visit can get off track if the wrong information is given to the nurse or assistant—or even if correct information is given that is misleading about your concerns. For example, if you say "pain" when you are really worried about an infection, or if you mention "fever" when you have leg swelling after a trans-Atlantic flight. These symptoms might be things you are suffering from, but they are not representative of your true concerns.

PAPERWORK: THE FINAL HURDLE BEFORE THE VISIT

Perhaps the final opportunity to frame your narrative, to yourself and to others, comes when you are given paperwork to fill out. No one looks forward to this, neither patients nor doctors. It is safe to say that no matter how paperless the medical office of the future claims to be, people will always have to provide extra information before they see the doctor, whatever the medium. Usually, that paperwork comes in several varieties, each of which is a significant opportunity to present your story in a way that will get things off on the right foot.

One is *the list of your current medications*. In a previous generation of medical record-keeping, this was done on paper (and still is in some clinics): the list of medications in the record is printed out and given to the patient for updating. This presents a number of difficulties. Often, especially if we are taking a number of medications, we forget to bring them to the doctor, or we don't have a written list of them. Obviously it would be better if we did. There are plenty of books advising us to be organized when it comes to our health, and making us feel guilty if we don't. I agree with them—we need to get organized. But even if we don't bring all our pill bottles or information to our appointment, we can still find a way to convey useful, organized information at that moment when we are filling out that form.

The key is to use the context to our advantage. It might be that the paper medication form or the fields in the electronic medical record are only designed to accept certain kinds of information: name of the medication, dose, and how often we are supposed to take it. That doesn't mean, though, that we are only allowed to mention these domains when we participate in the documentation of our medications. Even if we don't remember our medications and haven't brought them with us, any of the following statements can still be important information.

- *Ever since I started taking that medicine for diabetes, I've been going to the bathroom an awful lot. Diarrhea.*
- *I heard on TV that blood pressure medicines can cause problems with virility and erections. Is that true?*

- *I take so many medications, I don't remember which ones they are.*
- *Is there any way of getting any better medicine for pain?*
- *I heard that some of my medications can be dangerous.*
- *I forgot to take my medications today.*
- *I'd like to limit the number of medications I take. How many of these are necessary?*

Why should these things be mentioned even if they don't fit between the lines of the paper form or the electronic medical record? First of all, our issues are the ones that matter. We should not delude ourselves that the contours of the electronic medical record somehow magically map out what people want to talk about. If someone's concerns don't fit into the fields, and they are not brought up at an opportune moment, they might not be talked about at all. Conversely, since there is a timeslot in the visit set aside for discussing medications, and this timeslot will more and more be given over to the clinical pharmacist, medical assistant, or nurse, we need to make our concerns heard up front in order for the doctor, somewhere down the line, to hear them.

To put it another way, the new electronic medical records are designed by people in huge faceless corporations who might not have put much thought into what we need or want as individuals. There might not be room in the note that the doctor types up to talk about our particular experiences with medications. In the rush to quality that I talked about in chapter 5, precious real estate in that note might be taken up with formulaic questions about things that might not matter or the evidence might not support. I am thinking, for instance, of the presence in some "quality initiatives" of questions about seat belts. Seat belts are wonderful, don't get me wrong, but I am not sure having doctors ask about seat belts increases the fraction of people who wear them. If there is a nook or cranny where our particular concerns can be taken into account, shove a wedge in. Whenever medications are mentioned, we should make it our business to bring up our medication-related concerns, even if they are not precisely related to the name of the medication, the dose, or how often we are taking it.

FINALLY: FACE TO FACE WITH THE DOCTOR . . . BUT WHAT HAPPENS AFTER?

After the secretary, medical assistant, or nurse registers the purpose for our visit and after our medications are listed in greater or lesser exactitude, we will finally have the chance to be face-to-face with our provider: an MD, a DO, a nurse practitioner, or a physician's assistant. And, as I have talked about before and will talk about more in the coming chapters, we need to focus on building a productive and healthy relationship with that person, for the sake of our own health.

It helps to have as much time as possible to solidify the relationship. Incentives matter, and as I will discuss later, we need to restructure our health care system to help doctors spend more time with patients. Right now, however, in the real world, we should not feel self-conscious about extending a visit when we need to. If we are on time, or we have come the fifteen minutes early that every clinic expects but doesn't always request explicitly, we should not let a doctor's lateness deny us the time we need to address the issues we came for, provided we have constructed a clear narrative to explain why these issues are necessary to address.

The visit itself often ends abruptly, and there isn't as much of a transition as there should be between the time spent in the room with the doctor and the time spent without them. These post visits are perhaps even more important than the visit itself. How much time is devoted to one visit between doctor and patient? As I spoke about in chapter 1, the average number of minutes differs from country to country. Let's say for the sake of argument, though, that a doctor visit lasts fifteen minutes and we have a visit with the doctor every three months—more frequent than some people see their doctors, to be sure, but certainly not out of the question for someone with diabetes or other serious, chronic health problems.

In a year with that doctor, then, we would spend forty-five minutes at medical visits—which represents a very small fraction of all the time that passes during that year, 8.6×10^{-5}, to be precise. Such a dimension—the ratio between the time spent at doctors' visits and the time spent in the rest of your life—is comparable to a hundred-thousandth of a second, or the dimension of a cell wall. Later, we will talk about how the healthy conversation can be extended from the four walls of the visit to your entire life and its relationship to health. For now, though, it's important to remember that your interactions with the assistants and nurses before the visit are not just preparatory; they are part and parcel of the health-care interaction. Similarly, what happens after the visit is not just a petering out of the conversations during the visit, or a following up of the resolutions, but an active part of your ongoing health care.

By the end of the visit, there should be a plan made between you and your doctor regarding communication you should have during the course of the year. Can you communicate by e-mail or Skype? If you are comfortable using social media with your doctor, is he able to use it with you? If the preferred method of communication is by phone, whom should you expect to speak to when you call the office? How soon should you expect a return call, and what are the situations when you should reasonably expect to speak directly to the doctor?

"WHEN SHOULD WE SEE EACH OTHER AGAIN?" IS THERE AN OPTIMUM INTERVAL BETWEEN VISITS?

At the same time these frequency issues are clarified, the interval to the follow-up visit should be discussed. How often should someone visit their doctor? The answer is not at all clear. Many of us use the phrase "annual visit" or "annual checkup" without realizing that the history of this ritual deserves some examination. In a classic article, now more than a decade old, in the *Annals of Internal Medicine*, Christine Laine laid out the progression of doctors' thinking about visit intervals.[3] The first work to discuss seeing a doctor regularly for health prevention was published in the 1860s. However, the first widespread endorsement by public health organizations came in 1900, when the American Public Health Association publicized the necessity of the practice. Since then, doctors' opinions of the annual exam have undergone an up-and-down evolution, at first resistant, as Laine says, then enthusiastically accepting, and then—currently—carefully reexamining. The reexamination comes in the context of rethinking preventive medicine. It used to be thought that certain tests needed to be done like clockwork. The breast exam, the Pap smear, the prostate cancer test—all these things save lives, right? Plus you need to see the doctor just to get checked out: to have your heart listened to, to get your cholesterol checked.

But if you break things down, there's no iron-clad evidence supporting the necessity of these tests being done yearly. The breast exam saves no more lives if done every year than every two years.[4] The U.S. Preventive Services Task Force now recommends a Pap smear every three years.[5] And, as many people now know, the prostate exam and the prostate specific antigen blood tests are no longer regarded as matters of routine to be done year in and year out. There are even more examples for which there is no evidence one way or the other for the frequency at which tests or procedures should be done. "The optimal interval for [cholesterol] screening is uncertain," says the USPSTF.[6] Likewise for bone mineral scans, done to diagnose or check for low bone density, osteoporosis; the literature just isn't clear on how often these tests should be done.

Similar to the case of bone scans, there are many tests, procedures, and parts of the physical exam for which it just isn't obvious from the literature whether there is an optimal interval. The compromise might seem to be an easy one: do them regularly, at some round number of months, such as a year. Except the world has not yet seen a test or a procedure without a possible downside. Even a "routine" blood test is never routine, since it can increase the anxiety of the person tested and lead both patient and provider into a potentially endless spiral of ever more complicated tests and treatments when insignificant lab abnormalities are taken as harbingers of something terribly serious.[7]

What about the very foundation of the doctor-patient encounter, the history, physical exam, and the conversation that forms the backbone of the visit? Laine puts forward a powerful argument for their necessity. Only on the basis of regular visits between doctor and patient does there exist a relationship where health problems can be addressed if and when they come up. Take the particular example of someone who suddenly develops bleeding from the rectum, and comes to find that she has no regular doctor whom she can depend on because she had never gone to see one. It's not just that the doctor she'll end up seeing is someone she doesn't know, but also that it takes a certain amount of effort—"activation energy" is the term in physics—to surmount the institutional barriers that accompany anyone's first visit with a doctor. You don't want to confront such a hill if you are taking care of an ill friend or family member, all the more so when you are taking care of yourself. So seeing a doctor regularly is a way of laying the groundwork for future needs, says Laine.

But what interval is necessary to make this happen? Is it enough to chat every year on the phone, or is every six months more appropriate? What if an in-person visit is planned—how often is best? There's no way to know, because no one is likely to do a study comparing death or disease rates among people who see their doctors every six months, say, compared to every year. It seems unlikely that a practice, or set of practices, would consent to that level of variability in the visit frequency—or that patients would consent to it.

Laine's argument for the continuing necessity of the regular visit at some sort of arbitrary interval leaves out an important point. Her assumption, and that of many patients, is that the uses of the encounter between doctor and patient are static. Either the doctor "should" be using their stethoscope, or ordering blood for tests—because that is what doctors do! Or, on the other hand, we should see the doctor even if no immediate procedures or diagnostic tests are planned, because they might be indicated at some point in the future!

But there is a different, longer view one can take. The healthy conversation between us and our doctors can have its effects not in one visit, not even over a year, three years, or five, but over decades.

What are these effects? They are very concrete influences on our health but not the ones we are used to thinking about—the same ways we benefit from those around us in our daily lives. We benefit from many different kinds of relationships. Our friends, colleagues, acquaintances, and peers—we don't see them every day, but their words and actions have an effect on us. There are ways in which we mark our progress through life by our interaction with these important people.

OUR LONG-TERM HEALTH OBJECTIVES AS GOALS FOR OUR VISITS

Sometimes we can think of our health in medium- or longer-term ways that are more appropriate to the development of a long-term relationship. We would like to develop ourselves to our highest potential. That outlook can be applied to the improvement of our health as well. Our friends, in the Aristotlean sense, are meant to help us develop our best selves, and our doctors can do that too, together with us.

List the ten goals you want to achieve for your health—two in the next month, three in the next five years, and three in the next twenty years. Which of these do you need help with? Think of how you can enlist your doctor in the same way you might ask your friend or confidante for help. Perhaps you go to a friend for advice about an issue that has been worrying you, or just to tell her about an idea you have. Or you ask someone for an unbiased opinion about the course of action you are planning on taking. If you have made health goals and listed them, you can think of what sort of advice you are looking for from your doctor. It might be unrealistic to seek that kind of advice from one visit. Rather, just as you might only trust a friend you have known for a long time, you might have to invest in regular visits with your doctor in order to build a relationship you can rely on.

I have talked about how to prepare for the visit, both the hurdles of the prelude and the intervals between visits. But how do we make the most of the visit itself? In the next chapter we'll concentrate on the answer to that question.

Chapter Seven

Make the Most of the Visit Through Mindfulness

I've talked about what we want as patients: a connection to our doctor, and a doctor who knows what she's doing. We also know what the usual functions of the doctor-patient encounter are: building rapport, information gathering, and patient education—or partnership between doctor and patient. But many encounters between doctors and patients end up as complete failures.

It is easy to say it's the doctor's responsibility to follow the best communication practices. And certainly there are ways in which the health care system, and everyone involved in it, fails us as individuals. We do want our doctors to be properly trained in medical school about the best ways to listen to patients and take their wishes into account, while still "acting like a doctor" and fulfilling our expectations for the most effective care.

However, it would be unreasonable of us to expect that all or even most doctors are aware of these expectations. Most medical schools still conform to a so-called "biomedical model," in which we patients, people, are treated as if they were hosts to a constellation of disease processes and little else. Some medical schools have now begun to focus on communication,[1] but they are still few and far between. Even those medical students who, through natural inclination or their college education, have a fuller, well-rounded appreciation of the entire patient, often lose that realization during the methodical specialization training of their residency, their years as a junior doctor.[2]

As doctors get farther and farther away from their training, they forget what it was like at the beginning of medical school, when they were most like regular human beings. They become more focused on the particular body of knowledge they have gained with their specialization, and more apt to see the world through that lens. It is possible to make thoroughgoing changes in our medical education system. But, for the foreseeable future, most doctors will have come out of suboptimal training modalities that follow the biomedical model.

CREATING EFFECTIVE COMMUNICATION IN THE EXAM ROOM

Short of altering the doctors we have in front of us, we can try to create a style of communication in the exam room that helps bring doctors around to our way of thinking. I can't say that such an approach has the imprimatur of scientific proof—not yet. Most initiatives to improve doctor-patient communication that have been published in the widely read scientific literature are either disease-focused[3] or don't involve techniques that can be utilized by the individual person.

Disease-focused initiatives are great, and some have achieved real, though limited, improvement in the process and outcome measures we discussed in chapter 4. However, these initiatives tend to require a multidisciplinary team: not just the nurse, secretary, or doctor, but also a diabetes educator, a nurse practitioner, or a pharmacist. This is how modern medicine works; for example, the patient-centered medical home that I'll talk about later assumes that a group of professionals will be working with us every step of the way. However, changing the orientation of the group is too much to ask of a single individual. Indeed, concerns have been raised about the PCMH (Patient Centered Medical Home), that it places too much attention on the coordination of specialists, and not enough on a patient-centered attitude.[4]

Similarly, the Patient Protection and Affordable Care Act of 2010, more popularly known as Obamacare, mandates the creation of Accountable Care Organizations (ACO). These organizations are meant to provide incentives to groups of health care providers that take care of at least five thousand patients. Strict government regulations govern whether a group can call itself an ACO, and how much money an organization should save—that is, how much it should reduce costs—in order to share in the savings. This might remind you of the late, unlamented health maintenance organizations (HMOs). However, there is a crucial difference between an HMO and an ACO. While the insurance companies were in charge of reducing costs in the HMO system, it is the providers themselves who are penalized or rewarded for savings in an ACO.

Whether you are part of an ACO, a PCMH, or another part of the alphabet soup, you don't have much control, during the visit, over the communication practices of the whole team at once. The best you can do is to make all the circumstances as good as possible, both by making yourself ready before the visit, and by making yourself ready at the visit itself.

You have to be ready both emotionally and intellectually, but prepared to take the other person, the doctor, into account. This requires taking special steps in four different domains we will focus on in this chapter: *being mindful, centering on the visit, keeping an eye on the agenda, and being fully aware of the other's role.*

We talked about mindfulness in chapter 1, and its two components: self-regulated attention (awareness of one's own thoughts and feelings in the present moment) and orientation, the continuum of experience. Now we will specifically talk about the feelings and thoughts that one might have during a visit with the doctor, and how the doctor might respond to them. Centering on the visit and being fully aware of the other's role requires that we understand how the partner—the doctor—receives and responds to what we say.

HOW THE DOCTOR MIGHT RESPOND

We are all familiar with the "deer in the headlights" feeling that many people experience when they go to see the doctor. That feeling comes from patients being given too much information too quickly, as though having to drink medical information from the provider's fire hose. But the feeling also comes from being in a situation with poor communication. There is scientific literature trying to understand how we and our doctors assess the quality of communication during a visit. We can use this literature to advise ourselves on what to do in a visit.

The field of doctor patient-communication is still, after thirty or so years, in its beginning stages. Some scales and coding systems are standardized and widely used; however, in many studies, the investigators involved tend to fashion a system of communication and behavior description that, while similar to other studies, cannot really be compared to them precisely. In addition, much of the scientific work on patient-doctor communication is done in various settings, with different kinds of people, using a variety of methodologies. All this means that for the casual reader—whether patients or doctors—to understand the conclusions of the literature, it's necessary to get a 30,000-foot view that a communication review can provide.

Unfortunately, the most recent review of doctor-patient communication in the primary care office is about a decade old.[5] More contemporary are a series of articles done by Mary Catherine Beach, a mentor of mine at Johns Hopkins, and colleagues, concerning people with HIV seen by their regular doctor. Though these reviews are done in a specific population, they can be usefully generalized to the situation of anyone who sees a doctor, even if they do not have HIV/AIDS.

The methodology of these "ECHO" results, the name given to the larger study of which they are a part, is so simple as to be surprising: why hasn't anyone done this before? Doctor visits by these people with HIV were recorded and transcribed by a research assistant. Thereafter, various kinds of coding systems have been used to understand various aspects of those visits. The most frequently used kind of coding system is called the Roter Interaction Analysis System (RIAS), developed by Debra Roter of the Johns Hopkins School of Public Health in the 1970s. The system codes each utterance (i.e., something said by the doctor or the patient) into any one of forty-one categories, such as "Gives compliment," "Shows approval," or "Shows criticism."

Two types of categories in the RIAS system deserve some further explanation: "open-ended" and "closed-ended" questions. It has long been known that doctors often use closed-ended questions,[6] for example, "So you are here today to discuss your blood pressure." In response, it has been recommended more than once that doctors make an effort to use "open-ended questions"—for example, "Tell me please about the reason you came to see me today."[7] These types of statements, among others, are classified in the analyses used in the ECHO study.

This study has yielded research on a number of topics, including how doctor stress relates to communication; missed opportunities to provide empathy in the doctor-patient encounter; and the role of cultural distance as an explanation for disparities—that is, how people from different races or ethnicities with HIV receive unequal care.[8]

But I want to focus on an interesting, very recent finding that can help us understand what it means to *focus on our agenda with the doctor* and to *pay attention to the doctor's role*. This study, again done among patients with HIV and their doctors, looked at opportunities for doctors to display empathy and how they missed those opportunities.[9]

Missed opportunities for empathy have often been addressed in the literature on communication. Empathy, in the context of the doctor-patient communication, means knowing how to respond to emotional cues. Here is the way empathy might be demonstrated in a visit with the doctor:

You: I am really having an awful lot of pain and I wonder if it's ever to get any better.

Doctor: That's terrible—I'm sorry to hear that. I hear that you're in a lot of pain and I want to help you.

Now, like any other kind of response, there are authentic and inauthentic versions. Not every expression of empathy is convincing—in fact, emotional expressions on the part of doctors that are obviously fake can turn patients off. As one writer puts it, "a physician is clearly unable to comprehend and understand a patient's suffering and concerns while exhibiting an artificial empathy."[10] More than that, artificial or feigned empathy can deny the doctor the benefits of true empathy, which can accrue when they manage to imagine themselves into the other person's position.

However, even though fake empathy may be better than no empathy at all, at least it shows that the doctor is trying. Most often, in contrast to the exchange above, we get the following:

You: I am really having an awful lot of pain and I wonder if it's ever to get any better.

Doctor: How much is your pain on the scale of 1 to 10?

You: Um, it's pretty bad, I guess it's a 5 or 6.

Doctor: Where is it usually?

You: In my right side.

Doctor: How long does it last?

You: About half an hour or so, several times a day.

And so on. The doctor is focusing on the nature of the pain and hasn't recognized its importance to you. This is more evident in person than on the page, as the brief exchanges above do not capture the nonverbal aspects of the interaction with your doctor that signal empathy: the "back-channel" statements that signal that someone is listening to you ("uh-huh," "go on") and the attentive bending forward or receptive posture; the careful note taking.

How does it happen that doctors, who see pain every day and presumably understand the effect it has on people, do not—or cannot—empathize with you when you come to them reporting pain? Is it a failure of training, perspective, or incentive?

WHY DO DOCTORS FAIL AT EMPATHY?

They fail because of a little of all three (training, perspective, and incentive), of course. As Anthony Suchman pointed out in a seminal paper on the topic of empathy,[11] doctors are highly educated regarding the diseases that we come to them with. They understand our diseases, on the whole, according to a biomedical model: if the scientific principles that lead to disease are understood, then a cure can be pursued. The point in this model is not how a person feels about the disease, her symptoms, or the course of treatment, but how the "disease process," apart from the individual, has its effect in the body. "Pathophysiology" is the watchword for this view of medicine: how biology works wonders, or wreaks destruction, within the human being.

Most doctors, however, are not trained in how to respond to our emotional cues. They know how to fit a disease and its effects within the biomedical model, but so often miss the signals that tell them how we feel. And why would they be able to catch them? These are phrases and gestures that must be captured on the wing, and if a doctor isn't in the habit of noticing them, they can easily pass unobserved.

The second factor behind the failure of empathy is perspective. All the training in the world can't make a jerk into an expert empathizer—at least that's what our intuition tells us. But is it true? Can education in empathy reach the people who wouldn't be interested in it anyway? I think that's hard to say, due to the characteristics of the literature and of medical education. Different personalities are attracted to different specialties, as is well known; surgeons are by and large not weepy emoters, and primary care physicians do not strut. That would suggest, on the one hand, that those who are attracted to a career in primary care medicine are those who are already cognizant of empathy.

But the literature suggests something different:[12] those who are already interested can improve their skills. That is, there are probably some hard-core doctors who won't listen, no matter what, and can't be reached; we have little hope of changing them anyway, and they probably represent a minority of physicians. But the run-of-the mill general doctor, whose personality is probably attuned to empathy—we can show them how to improve.

In the above mentioned work, Hsu et al. mention that 70 to 90 percent of providers fail to take advantage of opportunities to show empathy.[13] However, they point out that few studies have asked why doctors don't do so. Is it because they are uncomfortable with emotions, because they are too busy with other tasks, or because they don't feel there's enough time to respond? If we knew the answer to these questions, we could figure out the best way for us to interact with our doctors during the visit.

The authors first had to define what kind of statement a doctor should be expected to react to with empathy. They called this a cue. Cues included medical concerns ("I'm always worried about my weight"), what they called "logistical life problems" ("I'm in a really bad low right now because I was supposed to go back to work on the 29th"), death or illness of a loved one ("My auntie died. Had to make funeral arrangements") or family strain ("We separated. We are still trying to get back together.").

These are the kinds of statements that we are prone to make when we need someone to listen to us. And they explain why we might, on occasion, try to limit our conversation to the doctor to solely "medical" topics; we also know that pressure in our life can impact our health and how we talk about it.

The interesting part of the Hsu et al. paper comes in the analysis of the providers' responses to the patients' cues. They recorded five types of such responses: Doctors either ignored or changed the topic; dismissed or minimized the cue (as the authors of the article put it, "denie[d] the legitimacy of the source of the patients' concerns"); elicited further information; attempted to solve the problem; or actually provided, though in the minority of cases, an empathic response.

You will be encouraged to know that the most common response type was not to ignore or change the topic or to minimize its legitimacy, but rather to elicit more information—just the sort of thing we are very comfortable with doctors doing. This happened among 37 percent of providers. Even empathic responses, though they happened in a minority of cases, were not vanishingly rare, occurring in 22 percent of provider responses. What we should pay attention to, however, is the "problem-solving" responses, found in 25 percent of provider responses.

Hsu et al. found that in about three-quarters of patient cues (16 of 29— note that we are not talking here about a huge study of the kind found in trials of medications. Such is the fate of communication researchers!), empathic responses were not provided to these cues. However, in half of *these* cases, the providers did engage in problem solving. To put it in simpler terms, even though empathy was not offered, problem solving was attempted.

This is the way that we ourselves, in normal everyday conversation, might approach someone who is having a problem. We might ignore it, though we would prefer to believe of ourselves that we wouldn't. We might imply or say explicitly that the problem isn't legitimate. We might on occasion even express empathy the way we know we should!

What happens, though, if we offer to solve the problem of the person we are talking to, without showing that we acknowledge the emotional effect that the problem is having? It depends on the person we are talking to, of course, but in general people prefer to be shown empathy. Emotional satisfaction is important, even if it becomes evident through some other means that problem solving is going on.

The Hsu et al. scientific paper helps us with two of the four tasks I mentioned above that get us on the right foot with communication during the visit: being mindful and fully aware of the other's role. It helps us with being mindful because, in paying close attention to our doctor's responses, we can figure out how the visit is going. Part of mindfulness is the simple act of paying attention, which we might not do often enough even in our daily lives. How much more do we neglect to pay attention in high-stress, technical, potentially dehumanizing, and infantilizing encounters, such as our doctor visits?

BECOMING AWARE OF THE DOCTOR'S ROLE IN THE VISIT— AND OURS

The other task this article is relevant to is being aware of the other's role in the visit. Below I have presented a transcript of a visit which is much like the kind of visit we go through every time we see a doctor. Your task is to pay attention to the exchanges and come up with an accounting of where you would have pointed the doctor's attention in a different direction. What do you think this person should have said? How could the doctor have behaved differently? Go ahead, mark up the page. And keep in mind some of the types of statements we already talked about with reference to the Hsu et al. paper: empathy (expressing acknowledgement of an emotional cue), problem solving, delegimitzation, or ignoring. There are, of course, other kinds of statements you might notice as well.

Doctor: Good morning. How are you doing today?

Patient: Okay, I guess. There are a lot of things bothering me.

Doctor: What are they?

Patient: Well, you know, I guess everyone has home problems once in a while, right?

Doctor: Uh-huh. Can we talk about your blood pressure? It's 150 over 70 today, which isn't well controlled. Are you taking your medicine every day?

Patient [sits up straight]: Oh yes I am, doctor, sure.

Doctor: Good. Because you know that high blood pressure can increase the risk of heart disease.

Patient: I certainly don't want any heart disease. My sister had a heart attack at age 56. That was just a few years ago.

Doctor: I'm sorry to hear that. What medications are you taking now?

Patient: I'm on so many medications, and sometimes I don't think that they help my blood pressure at all.

Doctor: Are you taking your medications?

Patient: I am taking them regularly. Actually, can I get a refill today? I just ran out.

Doctor: [sighs] I really prefer refills to be done through my office, but I am happy to do it now.

Patient: I have one more thing I wanted to ask you, doctor. I feel really tired all the time. Sometimes I don't even want to get up in the morning.

Doctor: Let me examine you. Then later we should do some blood tests to make sure your blood count, thyroid, and iron levels are okay.

Patient: Sure, doctor. Should I climb up here?

Doctor: Does this hurt?

Patient: [cell phone rings] Oh, I'm so sorry, I should have turned that off. [Answers cell phone.] Yes? I'm with the doctor. You're saying that my son is sick and I have to come pick him up? But...I'm with the doctor and I have to work today! [Hangs up.] Oh, that is crazy! I don't know if I can get through the rest of the day!

Doctor: Um-hm. I'm going to finish the exam now.

Patient: What should I do? I feel like my pressure is really high and all the time my heart is thumping away like a drum. Is there some way we can make sure that I don't have serious heart disease?

Doctor: Well, we discussed doing the lab tests. Then, if none of those come back to show anything, it might be a good idea to send you for a heart test.

Patient: Oh, OK. I just want to know everything's okay.

Doctor: Well, we can tell you if any of this is due to a heart problem.

This example is not hard to parse. It features exactly the kinds of statements that were mentioned in the Hsu article. By now you should have highlighted those statements where the doctor was trying to solve the problem without acknowledging the patient's expression of emotions—the ones that could easily have been yours in a similar situation. There were a number of statements in which the doctor failed to empathize, and others in which the doctor was trying to solve a problem even given the lack of empathy.

However, you might have failed to highlight another group of statements: the ones the patient made. There were many parts of the dialogue above where the patient could have made important though unobtrusive moves to emphasize the important aspects the doctor was missing. We don't often think of our role that way. As I mentioned earlier, there are a number of books that talk about the patient as passionate self-advocate. That's a fine role, and if that works for us, great. But we are not always able to assume such an active advocacy. Paying attention to the back-and-forth of conversation is easier for most people.

Let's take some examples from that conversation above. When the patient says, "What should I do," and the doctor responds with a litany of the tests that he or she is planning on running, what would you do in that situation? You could say something like, "What happens if the tests come back positive?" "How do you choose those particular tests?" "What should I do if the tests come back negative—are there more tests that you think we should do?" "What do you suggest I do about the symptoms in the meantime?"

Other ways to influence the course of the conversation involve pointing out subtly where the doctor might have missed the cues we have been talking about. "Um-hm. I'm going to finish the exam now" is a pretty closed-ended statement. One possible response to this might be to repeat what you said—"I really don't know if I could get through the rest of the day" or to ask the doctor explicitly, "What do you think?"

Of course, there are many moments in this dialogue where the patient, too, is guilty of less than ideal mindfulness. We might have made some of the same mistakes. Let's put ourselves in the patient's place. When we said, "There are a lot of things bothering me," we might instead have paid more attention in advance to which of our issues are more or less important, to frame the agenda in a useful way. This is a topic that merits a separate treatment.

Then there was the exchange with the doctor about the regularity with which we're taking our medications—compliance, as it is known in doctor-centered lingo. "I'm on so many medications," we said (again, putting ourselves in the place of the example patient), "and sometimes I don't think that they help my blood pressure at all."

That might be an honest statement but it is not as useful as it can be. Which medications are the problems with? How do we feel when we take them? Has it always been this way—since the first day we started taking them—or is this something that has only developed recently? And then, when the doctor asks us if we are taking them, we say we are—regularly. Coincidentally, we happen to have "just run out."

Medication refills work like this. If we see the doctor, and more or less on that day our prescription is sent to our pharmacy and we are scheduled to see the doctor again in some round number of months, it seems unlikely that our medications would just happen to run out right before our next scheduled appointment. Not to mention that asking for a refill while we are face-to-face with the doctor uses up precious minutes of time, both ours and theirs. We need to be clear at the beginning of the visit what our issues are with the medication, to guide the conversation onto a useful path.

Paying attention at the visit involves more than the aspects we have talked about here or the ones we will focus on in coming chapters. There is an entire encyclopedia of non-verbal "speech" that goes on during the visit—the postures you and the doctor assume at the beginning of the visit, when greeting each other, or when certain important discussions are going on. (For example, when you said in the dialogue above that you had taken all your medications, you sat up straight, as if to show yourself worthy of belief.) There's the way you and the doctor face each other, or don't; the manner in which the doctor interacts with the computer; whether physical contact occurs during the visit, either as part of the physical exam or not, and how you and the doctor react to it. Rather than an encyclopedia, we can actually call this collection of nonverbal interactions a Wikipedia, since either you or the doctor can edit it at any time and improve it through your own experiences.

Unfortunately, however, there's not all that much scientific research on nonverbal aspects of doctor-patient visits. Perhaps the resources required—video recording and analysis—are more intensive than the audio recording and transcription that are used in typical communication research. But the budget of the National Institutes of Health, which grants funds for "traditional" research on the biomedical model, is orders of magnitude larger than those of the Agency for Healthcare Research and Quality or the Patient Centered Outcomes Research Institute. Our priorities are out of whack, so, as I will point out later, understanding doctor-patient communication on a truly scientific basis requires a systematic restructuring of resource allocation for basic medical sciences.

We can all pay attention to the aspects of the visit to make communication better for us and our doctor. But what if we are too shy, unprepared, uneducated, unintelligent—or just plain intimidated? The next chapter will help us get over those hurdles.

Chapter Eight

How to Communicate Even While Intimidated, Limited, Uncomfortable, or Undereducated

GIVE ME MY DAMN DATA!

There are plenty of books out there to teach us how to boldly and proudly advocate for ourselves in the doctor's office. Doctors have held the reins too long, goes the story, and ignored what patients want and need. So it's time for patients to step up and ask for what we deserve. If there are medications prescribed, we should know how, when, and why. If there are tests to be ordered, we should have the results in hand. We should even have unfettered access to our medical records—this last expectation has a slogan attached, too: "Give me my damn data!"

Who would be so tone deaf as to deny people access to information about themselves? In the past, a patient often had to make a formal request for documents, and many offices charged patients for copying. However, with the development of new information technology and better security for electronic documents, doctors and hospitals everywhere are now becoming more open. If the "damn data" isn't quite as open yet as all that, it's now becoming a matter of course for patients to have access to a "health portal," where the entire record is available at a click.

This increasing expectation that all medical information be freely available is one of those historical phenomena that gather their own momentum until they snowball along, unstoppable by anyone's second thoughts. Nevertheless, there are two big problems with the assumption that our "damn data" will soon be widely available to anyone who wants it.

One is that the access is not as open as we would like to pretend. Not everyone is connected to the Internet day and night: only 68 million Americans are subscribed to an Internet service provider.[1] And, of those, there might be some whose access is only intermittent, (i.e., after the kids are in bed, late at night, at work). Intermittent access does not lend itself to thorough review of health records. Others must access the Internet only in public places such as the library, where access to secure sites may be limited or restricted altogether.

What about all the millions of Americans, nearly 55 million of them, or 22 percent of the adult population, per the Pew Foundation, who don't have any regular Internet access at all? When we talk about opening up health records, we are leaving those people out, or worse yet, deluding ourselves that they are included while leaving them dependent on Internet-connected people. And methods for providing access to health records for these "unconnected" adults are still reliant on formal requests and photocopying, which is not always offered as an option.

While the Internet is important, I don't think it's the be-all and end-all of communication between doctors and patients with regard to access to personal records and medical information. Like any other technology, there will be some of us who are not accustomed to using it—and thus what is supposed to be a conduit to a new age of open data might become yet another barrier to our relationship with the doctor.

BARRIERS BETWEEN US AND THE DOCTOR

There are many of us who encounter our visit with the doctor as a series of such barriers; access to records is just one of them. These can be personal barriers, as we have discussed above: the harried or short-tempered receptionist, the glib nurse, or the dismissive doctor. Or personal barriers can go by other names, if we are dependent on family, relatives, or other care-givers to access information for us. Then there are barriers of culture. We might have to take a long time explaining to the doctor why we aren't eating this month: no, it's not a random whim or a new fangled diet, but Ramadan. Or, yes, we have a big dinner Sunday after church. Perhaps we speak a different language more comfortably than we do English.

Perhaps the most common barriers are the different ways we and doctors think and communicate about health. It is easy to chalk this up to linguistic difference, because that is a factor as well. We call it bronchitis, for example, and our doctor calls it a viral upper respiratory infection. We come in talking about a funny feeling under our breast bone, and the doctor immediately puts it in the box labeled "chest pain." Or, conversely, the doctor has something in mind for us—for example, a test to catch early signs of colon cancer—and we don't fully catch her meaning because the words just aren't familiar (how many of us really understand the words "screening test"?). Doctors often use jargon they were taught in medical school, forgetting that most patients have not attended medical school themselves. Despite efforts to get doctors to explain concepts in "laymen's terms" many doctors simply don't know how, or don't want to, so they can better display their superiority in their field. Other times, they simply forget their audience and blow through terms that they know very well, but don't realize are not common terms.

BARRIERS TO COMMUNICATION IN THE HOSPITAL

Obviously, however, these differences in understanding words often reflect underlying differences in how we understand our body and our symptoms and their relation to our health. To illustrate this gulf and why it's important, though often bridgeable, I'll talk about a study I did a few years ago when I was a resident, a junior doctor at NYU.[2] The methodology was simple: I walked into patients' hospital rooms and, with their consent, asked them if they knew the reason their doctors admitted them to the hospital. I then recorded the reason they gave, and compared it to the reason for admission that the doctors listed in the medical chart.

While I had two collaborators who helped conceive the study and analyze the results—more on that below—the study personnel carrying out the data collection was all of one person, me. So I wasn't able to track down the doctors in person and ask them the reason they admitted the person to the hospital; I had to depend on the note in the chart. This was a weakness in the study. But, even taking this weakness into account (we know that chart reports are not always representative of what doctors think, and how these thoughts change over time), I still found the differences and similarities between what doctors and patients said to be revealing.

I shouldn't build huge edifices of theory on this study of mine. It was relatively small, comprising forty-six people. But it was novel, because not many people have asked patients before whether they have heard and understand the reason for their hospitalization from the doctor. Surprisingly, 11 percent could not give any reason at all. Of these five patients, for example, two had cancer diagnoses, not a kind of illness that you think would commonly go unmentioned by the doctor. In this study, I didn't go further into why these people could not give a reason, but you can easily think about instances where you or a family member might have been in a hospital; you could have speculated that one of the following might have contributed: too much going on at once, medical lingo, fragmented communication with too many doctors, and doctors themselves not being sure what the plan was at any time.

Of the remaining people I interviewed about the reason they were in the hospital, slightly more than half (52 percent) gave a reason that we thought agreed with the doctors' reason. My colleague and I, both of us doctors, determined whether the statements agreed or not. 37 percent of patients gave a reason for hospitalization that differed from their doctors' reason. We also looked at the kinds of disagreement between doctors and patients: sometimes the organ system (part of the body) didn't match in the statements, sometimes the type of problem with the organ didn't match, and sometimes the patient's statement was just too vague to compare to the doctor's.

What can we learn from this study, and does it apply to the doctor's office and not just the hospital? First, we learn that some of us don't understand what's going on in the hospital at all, or feel uncomfortable asking questions or giving our opinion about what we think is going on. If we have such difficulties in the regimented environment of the hospital, the problem might be similar in the doctor's office, where our reason for showing up to see the doctor and the talking points on the doctor's list can be quite different.

Part of the reason there might be such a lack of understanding, or at any rate, an inability to state the point of the hospitalization, is that it's not always discussed; other times, a doctor may not be clear in his or her intentions; still other times, patients don't ask questions for clarification. "You are in the hospital because you have an infection": a straightforward phrasing like that is not used often enough. And questions like, "I don't understand, doctor; what is the exact reason you're sending me to the hospital?" are not posed before a patient arrives at the hospital. Once there, patients, often being treated by doctors they don't know, may feel even less secure about asking questions; perhaps they're afraid they might offend someone or simply appear unknowledgeable about their situation.

The second lesson I would like to draw from this research, however, is more promising. Despite all the obstacles to communication between doctor and patient that I mentioned above, they saw eye to eye in our study regarding the reason for hospitalization a little more than half the time. And even in those cases when they didn't agree, I found, they managed to be on the same page regarding the organ system involved.

This means that there's hope. You and your doctor can manage to communicate. Even if you don't know your way around a health portal, there are still ways you can reach across the gap between you and your physician. Because we are human beings in relationships, we are expert in making connections with other people. We can use this basic ability to find common ground with our doctor. These connections start not only with the latest technology but with the common ground that defines our humanity, including the tools of our own cultures and backgrounds.

GETTING OVER THE BARRIERS: PRACTICAL CULTURE-BASED STRATEGIES TO BUILD CONNECTION AND COMMUNICATION

As in previous chapters, I would like to suggest some practical strategies to go about this connection-making. And, also as in previous chapters, the science here only gets us so far. There might be studies on patient-driven ways to improve communication, but they are not prominent in the scientific literature. At some point, even the scientist of doctor-patient communication needs to attempt to delineate commonsense strategies in the hope that they will help us talk to our doctors better.

Culture is a possible tool for leaping over the barriers between us and our doctors. Every group of human beings has developed strategies for connecting people. Since every one of us is born into a culture, we are already experts on such connections.

As a prelude to understanding the importance of these cultural tools, we should acknowledge how many doctors and doctors-in-training think about culture: as a source of gaps between groups of people and a contributor to worse health outcomes. Indeed, in their summary of methods to reduce cross-cultural miscommunication, Marjorie Kagawa-Singer and Shaheen Kassim-Lakha catalog the ways in which ethnic and minority populations in the United States lag significantly in multiple measures of health, including higher infant mortality rates among African Americans and Native Americans; higher maternal mortality among African Americans; and increased rates of end-stage renal disease in Mexican-Americans and African-Americans. This is not an exhaustive list. [3]

DOES CULTURE HELP US HEAL...OR GET IN THE WAY OF MEDICAL SCIENCE?

That these cultural categories are often confused with racial categories does not lessen the negative attitudes with which we and our doctors approach the notion of culture. Culture just gets in the way of the science of medicine, we might think.

However, as I have discussed above, we are realizing more and more how much so-called medical science is really based on slim or absent evidence. Treating mild hypertension with medications might do more harm than good; [4] getting screened for prostate cancer with a blood test might take us down a rabbit hole of unneeded tests; [5] and many of the "routine" tests proffered for years now by doctors' offices, for example EKGs, do not guarantee longer or disease-free lives. Thus, in most situations, doctors find themselves with a combination of incomplete information, professional custom, and competing values. This is where our values come in, filling in the space where incontrovertible science was long thought to be found.

In this same space, you can find all the things that make people what they are, one of which is culture. Kagawa-Singer and Kassim-Lakha, in their article, review the universal aspects of culture that contribute to the improvement and maintenance of health: Every culture, they say, strives toward "safety and security," "integrity and meaning," and a "sense of belonging." In identifying how a given culture specifies these particular goals (what is "meaning"? what is security? how do we strike the balance between them?), and the ways in which these goals are reached, the specifics of a culture are mapped out. And, specifically to our goals of improving health, disease and stress are experienced within a cultural context. Understanding that context can help us improve such circumstances.

I am oversimplifying a complex debate here. For as long as people have written about human society there has been a debate about the definition, importance, and meaning of culture. People vary in their willingness or ability to classify themselves into cultural categories, and can bristle when told to do so. Further, people can switch cultural categories, reclassifying themselves multiple times over a lifetime. And, last, it is not at all clear whether the path from "definition of culture" to "group sharing that culture" to "person in that group" is strong enough to hang causal relationships on. But that is why we have theories, after all, to organize our experiences and draw some conclusions—not necessarily that every conclusion be airtight.

Thus, even given all the caveats, culture can be a powerful tool to understand how you and your doctor can improve your communication. I think its use can be divided into two broad categories: how your culture is not relevant, and how it is.

DOCTORS' ASSUMPTIONS ABOUT CULTURE: DISCUSSING END-OF-LIFE CARE

Your doctor might assume, for example, that you are the kind of person who would like to make your health decisions independently. It's a common assumption that we need to be autonomous, even proudly so, as a reaction to many decades of doctor-centered medicine. But what if we are used to making decisions only in the context of our family and friends?

Often hospital patients and doctors have to discuss painfully difficult decisions about the kind of care the patients might want at the end of life. I know from personal experience that doctors are often frustrated when hospital patients insist that their families play a role in such decision making.

This is an instance where cultural assumptions get in the way, mixed with the unpleasant experiences of too many stressed discussions around the end of life. These doctors assume that the family usually interferes, or pushes decisions on the patient that he or she would ordinarily not take. Some of this attitude might be due to the pressures in intensive care units and some other environments, to "get the DNR [do not resuscitate order]"[6] (i.e., encourage people to decline resuscitation and ventilation in extreme circumstances), while the family would like the medical team to be aggressive in recommending artificial means of keeping the person alive.

I am not saying that resuscitation and ventilation are procedures everyone should choose for the end of the life; I would rather not have them done myself. But this is an example where the family and the patient can work together, with a medical team, in certain cultural circumstances, to find a decision that works for everyone. You might be the sort of person who does not make such decisions in the context of family or friends. But plenty of us do, and that is where culture comes into play.

USING CULTURE IN THE DOCTOR'S OFFICE

Similar considerations can be relevant in the outpatient clinic as well. For many doctors, the assumption is that one person's illness is best treated by involving only that person. If I have high blood pressure, the doctor talks to me about diet and exercise, limiting alcohol and salt, increasing fruits and vegetables. If those don't work, we might discuss a prescription. And that prescription is passed from the doctor to me, from one individual to another.

However, I go home and discuss my blood pressure with my wife—or, depending on who I live with, perhaps with my extended family. Like any family, we meet for meals, and what's in those meals can determine my blood pressure. More than that, I have ideas about what makes blood pressure better or worse, ideas affected by the beliefs of me and my family. Stress makes blood pressure worse—this is both a physiological fact[7] and a widely held health belief, at least among certain groups.[8] And how a person approaches stress is certainly affected by their culture: the beliefs, attitudes, and practices that we engage in every day.

Let's go back to the visit with this connection of culture and health in mind. One important cultural tool is people: the partner we live with, our family, sometimes even extended family or very close friends. The advice to bring someone with you to the medical visit is not new. But the reasons are usually advocacy oriented: the doctor might be incompetent or not have your best interests at heart, so have your husband nearby to speak up for you. Or they can serve as a secretary so you don't forget what's been said when you have your deer-in-the-headlights moment. However, another reason to bring someone to the visit is that the person you bring is part of you, in the largest possible sense. If making decisions is something you do with friends and family, it is likely a cultural activity; thus it would make sense to clue the doctor into that relationship by making it available to the visit.

So culture is not just what gets in the way of our encounter with the doctor. On the contrary, it can provide positive strategies to help us and our communities aspire to healthier behaviors. There are ever more examples of this in the scientific literature, which are usually discussed under the rubric of "community-based research":[9] we can get people around us, whole neighborhoods, to improve their health by implementing scientifically proven health interventions. But it works the other way too. Community-based interventions can help each of us, as individuals, convey the importance of our culture and community to our doctors.

To take a few ways in which such community-based intervention is being done: African American barber shops are used to get surrounding communities talking about blood pressure control; ultra-Orthodox wedding matchups have been coordinated through confidential computerized hotlines so that two carriers of Tay-Sachs disease do not end up marrying each other; employees in the same workplace (which, after all, is its own organizational culture) encourage each other to lose weight.

THE THREE PURPOSES OF CULTURE AND THE HEALTHY CONVERSATION: SECURITY, INTEGRITY, BELONGING

There are other ways in which culture can be enlisted in the service of the healthy conversation specifically, rather than just behavioral change in general. They can be built on the three purposes of culture that Kagawa-Singer and Kassim-Lakha laid out. For example, we can let our doctor know how we attain *safety and security* through our particular way of life. Who provides a sense of safety—our family, our partner, or a pastor? Or, on the contrary, is our culture, either the one we've been born into, the one we grew into, or the one we chose, one in which we do not actively seek out support outside ourselves?

"Integrity and meaning" might be a category that is less applicable in an ordinary visit with the doctor. But how we pursue that need through culture is relevant to our health. When do we think that we are doing the right thing? How do we try and find compromise between two conflicting courses of action? Here is one example that has come up more than once:

Doctor: How is it going, Ms. Davis?

Ms. Davis: I don't know. . . . My granddaughter wants me to move in with her.

Doctor: Is there anything wrong with that?

Ms. Davis: She says that I can't take care of myself, and sometimes I do worry about it, especially since I fell a month ago.

Doctor: What do you think about her offer?

Ms. Davis: Well, I don't know what to do really. I know she wants the best for me, but hope she's not trying to take advantage of me.

Doctor: What do you mean "take advantage"?

Ms. Davis: To take my checks, take my money.

We have an ethical dilemma. On the one hand, Ms. Davis appreciates her granddaughter's offer. On the other hand, she realizes there might be ulterior motives. What is the right decision? What would be the most honest way to relate to her own needs and those of her family? Which are more important?

Or think about when you discuss with a doctor the risks and benefits of a given course of treatment. You might have certain ways you think about yourself and your relationship with your world that inform your choice among alternatives. For example, you might not be "the sort of person who takes medicines," or you might be someone who realizes their limited tolerance for pain. If you are gravely ill, and the discussion is centering on goals of care for what time might remain, there are various approaches to these decisions that are rooted in culture. That's one reason such new services such as The Conversation Project (theconversationproject.org, an initiative to help patients and their families talk about their wishes for end-of-life care) are so important: they help us define explicitly what the approaches are to such difficult questions, not necessarily just on the basis of our own individual preferences and personalities (though that is legitimate as well) but on the basis of culture—what our families believe, what we have been raised to think is important, which groups of people we spend time with and what their priorities are to us.

"Integrity and meaning" overlaps somewhat with the last cultural function we will discuss, a sense of belonging. There are decisions in health care that have an impact on a person and their community: the stigma attached to mental health treatment, for example, or the disruption of work and family life that can occur if you need to regularly check in with an anticoagulation (blood-thinner) clinic to get your blood tested.

COMMUNICATION, CULTURE, AND COMMON GROUND

Culture is relevant to all sorts of health decisions. We should make sure that our home and family participate in our health decisions in a manner that's open to our doctor, so that we can all benefit from that glimpse into our world. But there is a positive influence of culture that is more direct: no matter what beliefs we have or practices we hold to, they can strengthen the common ground that is an important basis of the healthy conversation with our doctor.

Doctor and patient need to be able to relate to each other on a basic level in order that the visit fulfill the functions we mentioned in the very first chapter, and they need to do so as human beings who each come to the visit with their own education and expectation. Judith Belle Brown and co-authors, in an article from twenty-five years ago, explore how common ground needs to be reached on the basis of the common humanity of doctor and patient, in its possible diversity. [10]

Cultural common ground can be more important than people realize. A personal recollection: my father is a tax and bond lawyer who grew up in Philadelphia, went to various schools on the East Coast, and then in his thirties came to take a job in Louisville, Kentucky, where at least one client happy with his service gave him a ham. The only problem? My father is Jewish. He doesn't eat ham. Yet my dad went to some effort to find things in common with his clients in Louisville, even things he might not have been so interested in before. He started reading the sports section, which I believe was a new occupation for him. Similarly, because I am located in the Baltimore area, I have tried to know a little bit about the Ravens and Orioles so I can say something intelligent about Baltimore's favorite teams.

These are only trivial examples of topics that doctor and patient can share. Sharing common human experiences can provide a useful foundation to our relationships. It's funny to think of "breaking the ice" as it applies to a relationship with the doctor, but that getting-to-know-you applies to every relationship. I don't mean that you need to ask the doctor to share intimate details about herself, but you can ask, for example, where she went to medical school, how long she has been at this particular practice, where she lives. In so doing you can also help the doctor's relationship with you, doing some of the work she probably thinks about during the visit. As we have mentioned, one of the three main functions of the medical interview is building rapport: what more natural way to build rapport, for example, then to share stories about children, vacations, or relatives?

More seriously, all human beings have another source of common ground: we all know tragedy, and we are all going to die. So even if we don't have well-developed philosophies of life or approaches to how we want our lives to end, we all have firsthand experiences with the passing of loved ones, even with our own illness. It might take more trust than we feel we have in the doctor to ask, "What do you think you would do in this situation?" but you might be surprised. More and more, doctors are realizing that we want to hear, in certain circumstances, not just what the best evidence shows, but what the doctor thinks about the available choices as a fellow human being.

This is because so many health options are close to incomprehensible by the uninitiated. Should I agree to have surgery to limit the size of my stomach—bariatric surgery? On the one hand it can eliminate obesity with its attendant negative health effects, including diabetes: it's one of the only known cures for diabetes, the other cure being transplantation of islet cells, the cells of the pancreas that make insulin. On the other hand, bariatric surgery is a major surgical procedure with risks of death, complications requiring additional surgery, and failure—that is, some people who have bariatric surgery do not reap the hoped-for benefits.

The elements of medical decision making are complicated, multiple, and interlocking. Those of us, both doctors and patients, who are particularly invested in a certain vision of that decision making tend to see only one part of it—like many veterinarians examining a single huge elephant. Those who believe in evidence-based medicine are sure that all decisions, if founded on the best evidence, would become more legitimate and thus easier to make. Those who believe in the extreme version of patient-centered medicine would say that each of us ought to be prepared to make that decision for ourselves.

Yet none of these ideologies can completely bridge the gap between the patient with the doctor and the decision that has to be made. That is why some of us reach out, whenever possible, to the doctor, to find out what he or she can recommend to us as human beings. The evidence can say one thing or another, but what would you want for yourself when all is said and done? or for your mother or husband? If our doctor is evasive when we ask such a question, it might be because of systematic flaws of medical training, which make doctors think that they must not approach such questions as an everyday person would. These flaws deny the doctor the use of the powerful common ground that our shared humanity offers, and deprives them of an approach that might help us, their patients, in decision making.

COMMUNICATION, COMMON GROUND, AND END OF LIFE: REVISITED

We know from the literature about end of life decision making that doctors often want less invasive plans for their own end of life than those they might recommend to their patients.[11] This is not because they don't want to reveal such options to their patients, but because everyone thinks differently about themselves than about someone else. We are all most intimate with our own interests. It could be that doctors recommend a range of treatment options to patients and families at the end of the life because they don't know us. They mistakenly think that if we aren't offered the most intensive, technological, and invasive options, we might think the doctor doesn't care about us.

It is on that level that we need to find common ground with our doctors during decision making, by asking them what they might do as a nonprofessional in such a situation; by talking to them about what we find important in our lives, asking them about what they find important, and sharing experiences about implementing those priorities in the sensitive context of end-of-life decision making; and by encouraging and expecting doctors' display of emotion in such fraught circumstances.

On the basis of such common ground many aspects of the visit might change: the treatment alternatives proffered; the rapport between us and the doctor; and the personal relationship we have with each other that we can build on over time.

COMMON GROUND IN EVERYDAY CONVERSATIONS WITH OUR DOCTOR

Common ground doesn't always need to be used only in addressing decisions of major, life-changing significance, such as whether or not one should have major surgery. Every medical visit involves a myriad of smaller decisions as well that are not always evident to laypeople. Often these different categories of decisions are hidden—by design or accident—and their answers are assumed by the doctor. For example, take the following exchange:

Doctor: It looks like you have high blood pressure.

Patient: What should we do about it?

Doctor: Usually people can take one of a number of medications for hypertension.

Patient: Is there anything else that can be done?

Doctor: [quickly, with a lower tone of voice] Well, there are lifestyle changes—diet and exercise, of course.

Patient: How much do those help? That sounds a lot better to me than medications.

Doctor: [reluctantly] Okay, but your blood pressure is pretty high, and most of the time people use medication to control it.

What kind of exchange about treatments for high blood pressure might emerge from the common ground I have been talking about?

Doctor: It looks like you have high blood pressure.

Patient: I don't know about the treatments available and what you would recommend.

Doctor: Usually people can take one of a number of medications for hypertension.

Patient: What else can be done?

Doctor: Sometimes people can work on their diet and exercise.

Patient: What would you do if you had high blood pressure?

Doctor: The medications can actually be associated with a number of adverse effects. I suppose I would try to get things in my diet and physical activity in line as much as possible so I wouldn't have to take medications.

This exchange won't happen with all doctor-patient pairs. Many of us would start blood pressure medication at the drop of a hat if it were the thing that our doctor recommended—that's why it pays to have a healthy dose of skepticism with regard to medical evidence, since a recent analysis of a number of scientific studies found that, for example, medical treatment for mild hypertension doesn't lead to health benefits.[12] But, like many other things I am suggesting in this book, being skeptical is certainly worth the effort up front, and might help us save the effort we often spend after the fact scratching our head about what was said during the visit: why are we taking these medications, and how often? Are there supposed to be significant side effects or is that just something that has to do with us?

But wait, we might say, we know how the doctor's office can put us immediately in deer-in-the-headlights mode no matter how many self-help books we have read and how deeply we believe in the necessity of self-advocacy. All these examples we've talked about are very well and good for people who are comfortable bringing up questions to their doctor. For most of us, though, that's completely unrealistic. We are just not that used to asking questions of our doctor.[13]

There is definitely a scientific literature that encourages doctors to "open up fhe floor" during the visit to questions from their patients.[14] But what can we do to get used to the habit of asking questions? Like anything else, if we are starting on a new practice we might try doing it little by little at first. Here are some "starter questions" to make the asking come easier with time.

Questions for the receptionist or secretary:

What is the best way to ask questions of the doctor outside a visit?

When does the doctor prefer to be asked questions during a visit?

Are there certain questions that are more appropriately asked of the nurse or assistant than of the doctor?

Questions for the doctor:

I have some questions about this diagnosis. When would be the best time to ask them?

How and where do you prefer to be asked questions?

How certain are you of the information you just gave me?

What's the chance that the treatment you are suggesting will work? Over what time period should it work, and how certain are you of that estimate?

On the other hand, what's the chance the treatment you are suggesting will not work? What is the chance it will lead to significant side effects?

In keeping with the communication skills we are already expert in within our culture, as people situated in groups of other people, our question-asking facility with our doctor is only as good as our question-asking skills in general interaction with other people. I tend to be somewhat nervous when talking to someone I don't know, and I get mild anxiety-type symptoms—fast heartbeat, racing thoughts. Or, for example, perhaps you forget your questions in the moment and need to write them down in advance. This is always a good idea, whether you get nervous or not; sometimes our memories fail us or we think of something during the visit or while waiting for a doctor. Writing down notes and questions before an appointment is always a good idea.

Whatever your difficulties with asking questions, there are multiple practical, real-life strategies available, from rehearsal, to writing the questions down, to programmed reminders, to role-playing with helpful friends or family.

While access to the panoply of medical information is right for some people, there are strategies and skills almost every human being has equal access to: communication with our fellow human beings as part of our natural cultural inheritance. Using communication strategies we have learned with other people to find common ground with our doctors can make decision making more human, and a relationship more possible even at times of illness.

Discussing the agenda is another area of the visit in which practical real-life skills that many people already have can be transferred to the doctor-patient context. We will devote the next chapter to that topic.

Chapter Nine

What We're Talking About: Negotiating the Agenda With the Doctor

YOUR GOALS AND THE DOCTOR'S: WHY DO THEY DIFFER?

Let's say that you and your doctor are approaching the visit according to the suggestions in previous chapters. You are both mindful of the importance of the visit, both centered on the visit itself, as opposed to the transitory difficulties you might be facing in the day of the visit. You have found common ground on the basis of the basic humanity that you share. And you are ready to get down to brass tacks—accomplishing what you had in mind from the visit.

Even if you see eye to eye with your doctor on the importance of good communication, the goals you might have for the visit might be different from the goals of the doctor. This difference can have many reasons, and seems so natural to most of us that it doesn't need explanation at all. Imagine, however, if we were in a similar situation outside of the health care context. Would we expect that a mechanic wouldn't repair a car according to our specifications, or the restaurant cook would not prepare the food we wanted?

Perhaps a better analogy is with education. You are sure that you have learned the material correctly but the teacher still gives you a "C." You go and complain. "I did my level best and performed well on the exam," you point out. "You did try hard," agreed the teacher, "but you didn't make the standards for a 'C.'" The teacher has his own standards, inculcated in education school and via colleagues, and he is not going to bend them for the likes of you.

As I have already pointed out, medical practice today is most often not based on the best available scientific evidence; that evidence itself, moreover, is riddled with bias and confusion.[1] But the doctor has her training and priorities—which tend to be different from yours. How can we understand a doctor's goals and bridge the gap to our priorities?

Let's take a quick tour through the process by which a doctor decides on goals for your health care. First there's the explicit part. Some approaches to patients and diseases were drilled into the doctor during her first years of training, as a medical student or resident (junior doctor). If, after several blood pressure readings, the average of the top number (systolic blood pressure) or the bottom number (diastolic blood pressure) of a blood pressure measurement are above 140 or 90, respectively, then high blood pressure is diagnosed, for which treatment with medications is usually recommended. Similarly, if the level of glucose in the blood is high enough to justify a diagnosis of diabetes, then there are criteria to determine to what extent the blood sugar should be controlled.

The measure used to assess such control, the hemoglobin A1C, has been connected in various studies to the risk of complications due to diabetes, including heart attacks, kidney disease, and problems with the eyes and feet.

However, this brief summary of standards for the treatment of blood pressure and diabetes glosses over very considerable controversies in both areas. As recently described in the *New York Times*, a new systematic review (detailed, scientific merging of results from previous scientific articles) casts doubt even on the potential benefit that pharmacological treatment of mild hypertension might bring the patient.[2] At the same time, controversy has raged for the past decades about what level of sugar control, represented by what numerical value of hemoglobin A1C, is appropriate.[3]

Nevertheless, scientific disagreements somehow become transmuted into commonly followed medical practice. At some point, the doctor is going to tell you that she has reached a decision—or, perhaps leave out the decision making entirely—and tell you that "this is what doctors do" for the condition in question.

Unless you are a health practitioner yourself, you more than likely have no such approach to the health conditions you are dealing with. You don't care about the numbers so much as staying healthy—preventing catastrophic health events like a heart attack or stroke, maintaining your ability to do what is important to you in life, avoiding pain, and trying not to fall into a rabbit hole of complicated, expensive, messy treatments that don't help. The entire list of the kinds of things we as patients want is only now being clarified with the science of patient-related outcomes.

HOW OUR PRIORITIES ARE DIFFERENT AND HOW TO RECONCILE THEM

You could, perhaps, be in that minority of people who do understand their wishes in the same way that doctors do. In any case, the way you order your preferences is probably not the same as your doctor's ordering.

And this is where the agenda comes in. Many books tell us to write down what we are interested in talking about when we come to the doctor's office. The doctor's list might look like the following for a patient with diabetes.

Doctor's Agenda:

1. check hemoglobin A1C
2. discuss compliance with medications
3. discuss necessity of insulin
4. talk about diet and exercise

Your agenda might look like the following.

Patient's Agenda:

1. Urinating a lot, dry mouth
2. Worried about family history of heart disease
3. Memory loss
4. Will diabetes get better or worse and how will I know?

Addressing one set of agenda items will help address the other set. For example, when someone's blood sugar is high, as can be the case with uncontrolled diabetes, dry mouth and urination tend to result. Thus, controlling the diabetes would lead to fewer episodes of high blood sugar, that in turn would be reflected in the hemoglobin A1C: two priorities checked off at one go. Similarly, if you want to know about diabetes getting better or worse, discussing methods to check blood sugar (of that hemoglobin A1C is one) will help answer that question. Notice that several items on the patient's list are not found on the doctor's list, which is not unusual. Memory loss, while it can be affected, or even caused, by high or low sugar levels, is not necessarily related to diabetes, and thus might not come up in the doctor's agenda unless you bring it up. And, while diabetes certainly increases the risk of heart diseases—it is considered by many doctors to be the equivalent of disease of the coronary arteries—discussing diabetes does not perhaps answer explicit questions about the role of family history.

Just as important as the explicit agendas are the hidden concerns of doctor and patient. You might not be ready to talk about alcohol use or smoking explicitly during the visit, but they are certainly concerns on your mind. If you have a terminal illness, or know someone who does, the doctor might not be ready to bring up the goals of end of life care, though such a matter might be weighing on her during the entire visit.

Moreover, what you and the doctor think you might want to cover at the beginning of the visit might change during the visit; you might discover information, a diagnosis, or a treatment plan that upends the priorities you came to the appointment with.

This is why agendas should be discussed at the outset—not just because your and the doctor's priorities are different, but because they can change. In fact, for the past twenty years or more it has been recognized that agenda setting is a necessary part of the medical visit, but it is done quite rarely.[4]

AGENDA SETTING: MORE HONORED IN THE BREACH

How often is agenda setting done today? Using the transcripts of encounters between people with HIV and their doctors—the ECHO trial I mentioned in chapter 8—I looked for agenda-setting behavior at the beginning of the visit. I found that, of sixty-six encounters, only in one was there a discussion of patient concerns or priorities by the physician, with the phrase, "Tell me, is there anything you want to discuss today, in particular?" When I read that phrase, I wanted to reach out and shake the hand of the doctor who used it.

Most of the time, however, in forty-one of sixty-six encounters, the practitioner used a general opening question (e.g., "How are you?"). That phrase is used often enough in normal society as a common opener. But in everyday life we know that the phrase has many possible meanings: sometimes the phrase is meant more or less literally (i.e., as a query about our well-being), sometimes it's an automatic greeting without a question being meant (an equivalent to "Hi"), and sometimes it doesn't mean anything at all; it's an automatic space filler.

While we are familiar with ambiguity as part of the conversations of everyday life, a general opening question from the physician at the visit can be misleading. The doctor might be using the general opening question just as anyone else would in a social encounter, or she might be trying to get specific information from the patient about what he or she is doing. It might not be clear to you what the question means. Thus, it's not surprising that in most cases I looked at in my research study, the patient responded to the doctor with a general statement in return (e.g., "I'm doing fine."). In only a minority of cases did the patients respond with a particular complaint.

Perhaps these two research findings are connected. When it's not clear how the opening question is to be interpreted, the doctor might think that your complaints have already been asked for (How are you doing?" "Fine!"

Oh, okay, thinks the doctor), while you might be wondering when he is going to ask you specifically about your reasons for the visit. The ambiguity of the opening exchange might give the physician implicit permission to glide past agenda setting.

Why else might the doctor not ask us what we want to discuss? As I previously discussed regarding the reasons that might underlie a failure to communicate, it might have to do with education, personality, incentives, or a combination of all three. The doctor might be so consumed by what she finds essential (get the lab tests! control the blood sugar! normalize the blood pressure!) that she forgets that the person sitting in front of her has his own priorities. It is assumed that you, the patient, are a bundle of symptoms and diseases—and that those, not your own concerns, are the proper matters for a biomedical approach.

INCENTIVIZED AGAINST AGENDA SETTING

There are systematic aspects to the training and cultural conditioning of doctors that might also make it difficult for agendas to be discussed.

The priorities of biomedical orthodoxy often also determine the incentives under which doctors operate. As I have mentioned before, if we encourage doctors to improve the quality of their own practice, or the hospital practice they operate in, we are implicitly emphasizing measures that can be easily reckoned and compared with those of other practices. However, by the very nature of human beings, their individual complaints might not be susceptible to measurement according to some widely accepted scale. "I am worried about whether my diabetes is going to get worse" is not something that an electronic medical record knows how to record, or quality monitors know how to mark off on a checklist.

CAN WE TRAIN DOCTORS TO DISCUSS THE AGENDA?

Despite these difficulties, the literature provides some solid evidence that discussing agendas can improve the outcome of the medical visit. When patients and doctors are on the same page regarding the topics to be discussed at the medical visit, satisfaction improves on the part of the patient. [5]

Are there potential minuses to discussing an agenda? Perhaps such negatives are why doctors avoid it—or haven't been trained to do it—and why some doctors might think it unseemly to bring up their concerns explicitly. Doctors might be afraid that explicitly asking patients about their concerns, the first step to negotiating an agenda, might open up a Pandora's box of complaints.

We don't know whether this is true. It could be: if a patient feels free to talk about what is bothering her, she might bring up more complaints. We all know people like that. On the other hand, doctors addressing patients' complaints at the beginning of the visit might be a time-saver, helping doctors and patients avoid the dreaded "doorknob questions": "Oh, I meant to ask you one more thing." We don't know one way or the other.

We also don't know yet whether educating doctors to discuss the agenda with us at the beginning of the visit improves its efficiency. When a study recently published in the *Journal of General Internal Medicine* used such an educational initiative, the frequency of agenda-setting behaviors among doctors increased but there was no improvement in patient satisfaction or any significant change in the number of complaints in the visit.[6] It's unclear why this is the case. Perhaps people are not used to negotiating their agenda with the doctor, and don't know how to react when the doctor attempts it. As a doctor myself, I have had more than a few exchanges like the following:

Ms. Smith: Hi Dr. Berger, how are you?

Me: Great! What do you want to talk about today?

[pause]

Ms. Smith: [uncertainly] Well, I guess you are the one who wanted me to come in.

Me: Sure, I have things I want to talk about with you, but it's important for me to know what you want to talk about.

Ms. Smith: Nothing.

[The visit proceeds, and then Ms. Smith has some matters that she remembers a few minutes before the visit is due to close.]

This is frustrating—not just for doctors, but also for patients, because their concerns end up not being addressed. Perhaps there is not a widely held expectation that you and your doctor can explicitly discuss the way in which the visit is going to go. After all, many kinds of interactions in our lives share this lack of agenda-setting. We have a meeting with our children's teacher and are not sure how the conversation is supposed to go. Even casual social situations make us awkward because it's not clear to us what we are supposed to say. Not all social interactions need to be scripted, but sometimes what lies beneath the surface needs to be made explicit by identifying the agendas, both stated and unstated, of both parties.

HOW CAN WE LEARN TO ADDRESS THE AGENDA?

So how do we make sure that the agenda is addressed during our visit? First, we have to bring it up; then, we have to let the doctor bring it up; we have to negotiate the balance between our two agendas; and we have to see them through to the end of the visit, making sure that the items on our agendas are actually covered.

Bringing up our agenda means mentioning it explicitly, using any one of the following phrases, or whatever works for you:

I have some things I want to discuss.
There are some things bothering me.
I brought a list of things to talk about.
Can I go down my list?

It would be a tone-deaf doctor who wouldn't welcome someone who had prepared a list of topics in advance. But, on the other hand, it's common to find that doctors do not explicitly tell us what they are going to talk about during the visit. So it is also our job, in the doctor's office, to make the doctor's implicit agenda explicit. "What is on your list to talk about, doctor?" might be a phrase that many of us would have difficulty bringing to our lips, but there are other more palatable alternatives. "What do you think we should talk about today?" is another possibility, or simply, "What's on the agenda?"

Once you and your doctor have gotten that far, it's time for the hard part: negotiating between your agenda and your doctor's. That is not the only alternative. Perhaps the most common approach to conflicting agendas is still to let the doctor hold the reins and take control of the visit, with us trying to get in a word where we can with our own concerns. And then there's the other end of the spectrum, where we take over control of the visit without regard to what the doctor would like to cover.

If you assume, however, that balancing both parties' concerns is common sense, and perhaps even saves time—though we can't be sure of that on the basis of scientific evidence—how can we bridge the gap between our agenda items and the doctor's? Bridging this gap is another area where common difficulties in the doctor-patient visit outrun the science. No one has done a study comparing ways in which we and our doctors can negotiate.

This is not to say that the scientific literature has not addressed the topic of doctor-patient negotiation in general. For example, twenty years ago, in an article in a family practice journal, Richard Botelho described the doctor-patient encounter as a negotiation. But while he gives a useful description of the aspects of the medical interview that we have described elsewhere, he does not provide any recommendations about how to communicate. [7]

SPECIFYING WHAT WE WANT FROM THE DOCTOR

If we are to do so, we need to clarify, first, what the kind of things are that we patients ask for during the medical visit. R. J. Kravitz and co-authors did just that in 1999 in the *Journal of Family Practice*.[8] In order to understand negotiation in office practice, they created a classification system called the Taxonomy of Requests by Patients (TORP).

Why is such a taxonomy necessary? The authors point out that people come to the visit with different sorts of ideas: not just requests but also desires and expectations. Desires can be defined as wishes regarding medical care, while requests are desires that are explicitly expressed; expectations are wishes that are not explicitly expressed. Unfortunately, some of the common phrasing that we and our doctors use to discuss the agenda—some of which we have already made use of—confuses this distinction.

Kravitz and co-authors, in developing their taxonomy of requests, defined them as "the patient's hope or desire that the physician provide information or perform action. Requests may be expressed as questions, commands, statements, or conjecture. Most questions are requests, except rhetorical questions ('Who do you think I am?'), exclamations ('You're kidding, aren't you?'), questions related to the mechanics of the physical examination ('Where should I sit?'), and chatting on topics unrelated to health or medicine ('It's sure been hot, hasn't it?')"

Based on hundreds of recordings of visits, they developed a classification of requests that includes two broad categories: requests for information (for example, about symptoms or treatments' about psychosocial issues, about physicians, about administrative issues) or requests for action (for example, about the physical exam, tests, treatments, referrals, or administrative matters).

This classification system was consistent among the authors: that is, there was good agreement among various people who used this system to classify statements of patients. They found that 98 percent of patients had a request during their visit, and that if these requests were not met, patient satisfaction was lower. This is just the empirical verification of common sense.

Not every patient statement at the doctor's office is a request. And not every request is clearly either for information or for action. Our asking for advice from a doctor, for instance, might fall into both categories at once. We might make requests without knowing precisely what we want. But the classification the authors give might be a useful first step.

BRIDGING THE LANGUAGE GAP

If you are coming to a doctor and you want information, you are going to have to bridge the gap between the language of the ordinary person and the language of the doctor. As I mentioned in connection with my research in the hospital, we and our doctors usually do not express ourselves the same way when it comes to describing our medical concerns. You say you have back pain; the doctor says you have sciatica. You say you are worried about a heart attack because of your chest pain, the doctor says you have gastroesophageal reflux disease. You might want information about how your diabetes is going to progress and what you can do about it, while the doctor tells you that there is a certain range your blood sugar should be kept in.

When you and the doctor aren't seeing eye to eye in the terms you are using, there are several ways to bridge the gap—or at least to make a detour around it. In some cases, as in the example of diabetes control, the doctor might not know what the specific connection is between the treatment he is suggesting and specific, positive effects on your health.

I have used diabetes as an example multiple times because, for our era, it is *the* disease—the chronic ailment that affects multiple organs of millions of people around the world. It also reflects the tenuous state of medical knowledge. Doctors still are in dispute over the proper range for blood sugar and whether more or less intensive therapy for diabetes will protect various organs of the body.

Staying with the example of diabetes, you might want a certain kind of information:

You: What range should my blood sugar be in for optimal health?

[While the physician answers with alacrity.]

Doctor: Anywhere from 90 to 130 when you are fasting—that is before you eat and drink—and 140 to 180 when you have had a meal.

This does not actually answer the question you were asking. You were not asking, "What are the generally accepted guidelines for control of blood sugar in someone with diabetes" but rather, "Where should 'my' blood sugars be controlled to? What numbers are the most advisable for me?"

This space between the guidelines of professional societies (internal medicine doctors or diabetes experts) and the questions of an individual patient are where the rubber meets the road for doctor-patient communication and shared decision making. This is a secret known to all doctors that have thought about it but too rarely realized by people who aren't health care professionals: there is often nothing magic about doctors' suggested guidelines. Why should blood sugar control be focused on the arbitrary limits 90 and 130, especially when doctors don't agree on where the hemoglobin A1C, an integrative measure of blood sugar over a few months, should be?

Because we don't know how to individualize blood sugar goals for our particular circumstances, we will need to work out a compromise with the doctor. And since the doctor, by dint of practice, is likely to be more familiar with appropriate blood sugar goals than we are, our compromise reached during discussion of the agenda is likely to be more in the direction of orthodox medical advice than our own preferences.

However, there are also going to be situations where we are sure that the right thing to do is something that the doctor thinks is inappropriate.

THE MOST DIFFICULT NEGOTIATION: WHEN WE DISAGREE WITH THE DOCTOR

The archetypal example here is back pain—another area that I, both as a normal person and a doctor, know something about. A few months ago, I got to participate in an exciting initiative that presages epoch-making changes to our medical system. The whole idea goes by the name "Less is More": and the meaning's in the name. Many things done in the name of health under our current perverted medical system, such as overprescribed and overused medical tests, do not promote health, but instead threaten us with harm and cost patients and our medical system more money. I'll address these systematic issues in detail in chapter 14, but the boulder we helped give a running start to is now rolling at full throttle down the hill.

A prime example of overprescribed and overused medical tests are those for acute lower back pain. A few months ago, as part of the "Less is More" intiative, I was part of a team that published an article synthesizing the evidence that supports imaging (CT scans, MRIs, and X-rays) for lower back pain without "red flags" (i.e., back pain without alarming signs that can portend infection or cancer).[9]

The results weren't good. Our American health care system spends hundreds of millions of dollars a year on these scans, and they don't work. Lower back pain without red flags, so-called "garden variety" lower back pain that accounts for the vast majority of back pain, most often resolves in a few weeks and does not reflect any serious underlying systematic disorder. Obtaining images is most often unneeded, because the procedures expose the body—in the case of CT scans or X-rays—to unneeded radiation; because the person, or the health care system, incurs unneeded cost that would be better used for other things; because they can worsen the anxiety of the person who is undergoing the imaging; and because they can send that person down the rabbit hole of test upon test, procedure upon procedure.

We all know how this happens. A "routine" MRI, say, is done for back pain. MRIs show a lot, every nook and cranny of the muscles and tendons: the soft tissue of the back. Some of what is shown is bound to be interpreted by a radiologist as abnormal, even if it might not have any connection to the symptoms of the patient. Perhaps that abnormality will prompt a doctor to refer that person with back pain to a surgeon. Where there is pain, an abnormality on imaging, a willing person, and a surgeon desirous of helping, a procedure might indeed come about. As we know, however, surgery is not a foolproof cure for the most common types of back pain without red flags. [10]

With my doctor hat on, therefore, I know that imaging should not be automatic in garden-variety lower back pain. But then as I carried a very large cardboard box, a moving carton, full of baby clothes from our basement to the third floor, something twisted out of place in my right lower back. I was attacked by short bursts of sharp pain. "I want an MRI!" screamed my brain several times during those first exquisitely painful thirty-six hours.

I didn't ask my doctor for one, because my doctorly instincts won out. I understand better now why people want them. They want to make sure that nothing is broken and nothing dangerous is afoot. The only way to provide those reassurances, however, is not with imaging, or blood tests, or even with the physical exam—it's with the conversation.

In most cases of back pain, doctors can't put their finger on any specific cause. Things get better by themselves. Surgery doesn't help much most of the time. Yes, you are a unique individual: but your garden-variety back pain is probably best treated the way it is for most people, with pain remedies, heat, and physical therapy.

Telling someone that their exquisite pain is best treated with simple workable approaches, misnamed "conservative treatment," requires some emotional capital as does any agenda negotiation involving procedures that we want to see happen but the doctor doesn't.

Thus, unfortunately, I can't tell you that there's a foolproof way in an individual visit to successfully convince a doctor to do something she doesn't want to do. Or, contrariwise, to agree to back off from a course of action that you think is unwise, but that the doctor is pretty sure needs to be done, according to protocol. More likely than not, you will acquiesce to what the doctor recommends; such is the inertia and the imbalance of the typical doctor-patient relationship. However, if you already have a relationship with your doctor, you might be able to negotiate about the actions that you and she do not see eye-to-eye about.

For example, regarding an MRI for back pain, you might say, "I understand that doctors do not recommend getting an MRI or another sort of a scan for back pain, but I am worried that something might be broken back there. Is there a way to check on something like that?" The doctor might say that such a scan isn't recommended, but then perhaps in return you could suggest another possibility: another sort of scan he or she didn't mention (an ultrasound, perhaps, can sometimes be used to look at soft tissue). Or perhaps the doctor, in response to your concerns, might be able to tell you that in fact there is nothing broken in your back.

These exchanges aren't all going to happen in the space of a fifteen-minute session. Negotiation doesn't only take place in a single visit, it plays out over the entire lifetime of the doctor-patient relationship. That relationship will enable the steps I have discussed in this chapter: making your and the doctor's agenda explicit, bridging the gaps between the terms we use, and negotiating a compromise to reach a shared agenda.

Besides compromise and the explicit agenda, our relationships with our doctors are founded as well on emotions. In the coming chapter I will discuss how your and your doctor's emotional resources can be used to put your relationship on a steady and productive, as well as healthy, footing—because if we can negotiate about medical issues, we can also negotiate about emotional concerns.

Chapter Ten

Acknowledge—and Use—Emotion and Motivation

HOW WE FEEL WHEN GOING TO THE DOCTOR—AND HOW THE DOCTORS FEEL TOO

Have you ever felt scared and intimidated when going to the doctor's office? There are many reasons why you might feel that way. The lighting is unforgiving, bringing to mind the interrogation scene in a movie; the secretaries are harried; the group practice consists of a number of doctors who are always busy and don't remember you; phone calls are returned with delays; and, once you make it to the doctor's office, the effect of the doctor's position and your uncertainty is to distance the visit itself from what you care about—which can be alienating and frightening.

So, yes, fear and intimidation, or just alienation and nervousness, are common accompaniments to a visit to the doctor. But we should also realize that the doctors we see have their own emotions that are present during a visit. One of my colleagues told me during medical school, "If you don't feel a little bit nervous every time you go into a patient's room for the first time, you're probably not paying attention." Nervousness is among the most benign emotions that doctors feel. They can be scared as well for the patient's sake, worried that their ignorance might put the patient at risk, distracted by many other commitments, distressed by potentially unpleasant or weighty social interactions, or just tired from work and the pressures of daily life.

Yet have you ever been at a visit with your doctor where these emotions were acknowledged? I have not, and many people I know have not, either. Conversely, in my experience working with and teaching junior doctors, I have found that a number of them are uncomfortable addressing emotion. The reasons for this are multiple: sometimes it may be because these doctors have not yet found their place professionally and think that demonstrating emotion will cause their colleagues to look down on them. Perhaps they are not centered enough on the visit to be able to incorporate their emotional experiences and interactions into the flow of their work, and those emotions throw them off guard.

The most visible emotions during the patient-doctor encounter are the ones that are easiest to notice in everyday life. Anger heads the list, and it takes a certain sort of personality, augmented by careful training, to know what to do when a party to the medical interview is angry—all the more so when violence is anticipated or threatened. People burdened by depression or significant psychosocial stressors can burst into tears when asked about their situation. Diagnoses and treatments can bring fears to the surface. Negotiating this territory requires nimble emotional reflexes.

Then there are the emotions that lie just underneath the surface and require active effort to be recognized by the parties to the conversation. Fear does not always bubble up to the facial expression or the tone of voice; similarly, nervousness, boredom, suspicion, guilt, and self-reproach also play their roles, like individual musicians in an orchestra.

CAN GOOD MEDICINE BE EMOTIONAL?

One common objection to recognizing emotions during the medical visit comes from the biomedical model. Medicine is founded on strict objectivity, as all sciences are (goes this logic). Involving one's emotional judgments in a medical decision, or in discussing the facts of the medical case, can skew the judgment of our doctors and make them less likely to use the best cognitive techniques at their disposal to reach a correct decision on diagnosis and treatment.

In a certain sense, this is correct. Emotion can shunt the thought process of doctors, and us, too, onto certain paths, where it might be more difficult to obtain the necessary wide-ranging view of a situation. The most publicized writing about this area has been done by Jerome Groopman,[1] but apart from his work, a considerable literature has grown up around the cognitive processes of effective doctors. Doctors and cognitive scientists are trying, with various degrees of success, to find out what goes on in a doctor's head when she considers the facts of our illness, and arrives eventually at a diagnosis and possibilities for treatment. There are many biases that can get in the way of this delicate reasoning. For example, availability bias refers to our inability to imagine situations that we have not been exposed to, or are not familiar to us. Doctors have a saying about availability bias: where there are hoofbeats, don't expect zebras. Sometimes, though, a zebra is the correct animal after all, and it is the bias—the inborn thought habits—of doctors that get in the way of making the correct diagnosis.

The concern is that involving emotions in the medical encounter can encourage the exercises of these biases. Frustration with a patient can make it more likely to overlook the full range of diagnostic possibilities. If we are fixated on one disease we are worried about, and get on the doctor's nerves, our doctor might be tempted to ignore the disease, or at least downgrade its importance. Acknowledging these emotions would be lending credence to them and detract from the strict empiricism on which effective medical treatment is based.

There are two responses to this critique. One is that emotion can help our doctors avoid these cognitive biases. It is a widely recognized tenet of professionalism that doctors maintain for us "unconditional positive regard":[2] even when we are annoying with our pain complaints and insistent with our questions, we are supposed to be appreciated as the human beings we are, as part of the doctor-patient relationship. We must not be ignored. Countless times, in the heat of a busy clinic day, I have almost overlooked the complaint that someone has come to me with. It is only their obvious pain—in some cases, their refusal to back down—that has made me take notice. I am imperfect. It is my identification with a fellow human being, facing me in their chair, that makes it more likely to "keep a broad differential" (i.e., make sure I am not ignoring any likely possibilities).

However, there is an even broader critique that is possible here. The cognitive scientific model of thinking and decision making on the part of doctors and patients is limited by its foundational assumptions, like in many other sciences.

According to cognitive theories, doctors use two types of reasoning to reach a diagnostic conclusion. One method is heuristic reasoning, in which the doctor logically arrives at a conclusion after considering all available evidence. The other type of reasoning is more intuitive, in which the doctor makes a leap from a limited set of information, following a pattern, to reach an answer.[3]

Such a description of the cognitive work of doctors is misguided because it assumes that medicine is objective. There is a single medical truth identifiable in a given situation, and the doctor's job is to find it. This does describe some fraction of encounters. But more often than not, neither doctor nor patient leaves the encounter knowing what the reason is for the complaint. Even in those situations where a diagnosis is arrived at, often, almost a third of the time (as established by autopsies) the diagnoses are incorrect.[4]

This is not to say that the customary image of doctors—diagnostic thinkers who ferret out the pathophysiology at the root of the problem—is always false. It's that most often, the function of the medical visit is to fulfill the three functions (collecting information, building rapport, and education and discussion), not in service of objective truth, like a scientist would want, but to heal the patient. And healing depends on sensitive emotional navigation as much as objective truth.

In this way, medical decision making is much like any sort of cognitive function: it depends a lot on emotional cues. Without functioning emotional intelligence, it becomes very difficult to apply the heuristics and diagnostic reasoning to actual people.[5] Without emotional nimbleness, it becomes impossible to apply the theory of medicine to practice.

BRINGING EMOTION TO BEAR IN THE MEDICAL INTERVIEW

There is an important, positive example of how emotion should be brought to bear in the medical interview: not as an outside, extraneous tool, but as a basic element at the very foundation. I am referring to the practice of motivational interviewing.[6] Motivational interviewing is a tool that helps both parties to the interview discuss behavioral change. Its key elements are these:

1. It is not directive. Doctors tend to tell us what to do—You should stop smoking! You should lose weight! In contrast to this, motivational interviewing, as its name indicates, attempts to solicit our own reasons for our health-affecting behaviors. We might know that we should quit smoking but feel powerless to do so. Our weight is a problem but it's something we're just not ready to fix right now. So motivational interviewing does not tell us to do something, but rather gets us to open up about our thoughts.

2. It is supportive. The doctor properly trained in motivational interviewing knows not to criticize us for the changes we have or have not made. Sometimes things are outside our control. And, more important, unsupportive statements will not push us toward behavioral change any faster. The doctor is open to what we have to say about our experiences, receiving the information as data to help modify treatment now and in the future.

3. It is narrative. The doctor tries to ask, in open-ended fashion, about our experiences with the behavior we are struggling to change. These are not questions about particular sets of symptoms, but about the entire arc of our story.

An example of a conversation between someone and their doctor about smoking, not using the principles of motivational interviewing, might go like this:

Doctor: You're coughing? You must still be smoking.

Ms. Wilson: Yes, I am.

Doctor: You really should quit. Can I give you some nicotine patches?

Ms. Wilson: Sure, I'll take them.

With motivational interviewing put to use, the conversation might go in a different direction.

Doctor: I notice you're coughing. Can you tell me about your smoking?

Ms. Wilson: I'm still smoking.

Doctor: What do you feel about that?

Ms. Wilson: I feel awful about it. I know it's terrible for my body, and I feel so guilty that after all these years I'm still not able to get a hold of it.

Doctor: Why do you smoke?

Ms. Wilson: I think it helps control my weight. It really takes the edge off after a long day at work. I can feel the tension draining out of me with that first cigarette. Do you know what I mean?

Doctor: Sure, I hear a lot of people tell me that.

Ms. Wilson: But I really know I should quit.

Doctor: Tell me about the reasons you don't like to smoke.

Ms. Wilson: It stinks, it turns my teeth brown. [Laughs] I could sit here all day and list the reasons why smoking is bad for you. I know that it is bad for the heart and makes my cough worse. I know all that. I know what you doctors want to hear.

Doctor: But I would rather hear the reasons why you think it's bad for *you.*

Ms. Wilson: You know why I can't stand the smoking any more? I'll tell you the truth. It's because it's taken over my body. I hate the smell, I hate what it's done to my teeth, and I hate the money I've spent on it, but I just need to keep smoking cigarette after cigarette, like I can't help it.

Doctor: Do you feel like you're ready to quit?

Ms. Wilson: I know I should quit. . .

Doctor: Can you put a number on how motivated you feel to quit?

Ms. Wilson: I feel very motivated, like an eight out of ten, but I don't feel very confident at all.

Doctor: Why don't you feel very confident?

Ms. Wilson: Because quitting smoking—I know this from other people who have done it—takes a lot of effort and concentration. And since there is so much else going on in my own life, I can't focus on quitting smoking. That's why I feel that when push comes to shove, I won't be able to handle it. I know that's wrong, but that's the way I feel.

Doctor: I don't think that's wrong. What do you think are the next steps we should take? Are you ready to set a quit date?

Ms. Wilson: [hesitates] I don't know. . . . .

Doctor: You sound like you're not ready.

Ms Wilson: You're right, I'm not ready. I'm just so scared.

Notice the emotions that are brought to the fore in this discussion: fear, self-doubt, uncertainty, and lack of confidence—though she doesn't lack motivation. The provider elicits Ms. Wilson's story without pressing her to take any particular conclusion. The motivational interviewing serves as a wedge driven between Ms. Wilson's lack of confidence and her motivation to change, opening up a space where she can act when she chooses to.

Motivational interviewing has been found useful in a broad range of health problems.[7] Many medical problems depend for their improvement on behavioral change. If it's not giving up drugs or having safe sex, it's following a diabetic diet, taking medications regularly, finding support for depression, or participating in a regular exercise regimen to help with pain or musculoskeletal problems.

Even if no deleterious habits (poor diet, substance abuse, unsafe sex) are involved in the particular doctor-patient encounter, the emotional approach of motivational interviewing is still of great importance. Changing behavior can be fiendishly difficult, as anyone who has tried it can attest. Much of health care depends on changing behavior, however, whether it be incorporating new medications into your life; changing diet or exercise; avoiding other bad habits; or even attending a visit with the doctor and modifying one's lifestyle on the basis of that discussion. Thus, motivational interviewing, and the principles underlying it, can be relevant to any visit with the doctor.

RECOGNIZING EMOTIONS AND PUTTING THEM TO USE

Besides motivation and confidence in our own ability to enact change in our lives, there are many other emotions at play—as I have mentioned—in our encounter with the doctor: anger at illness, hope for cure, desire for a working, meaningful companionship, desperation, boredom, and fear. If we can recognize them, call them out by name in our own minds, we can train the circus beasts and have them do our bidding. By acknowledging doctors' emotions, and meeting them with our own, we can lay another sort of foundation for a healthy relationship.

But which emotions can be used to that end? Not every emotion is useable. How should we approach these emotions and put them to use?

HOW TO ADDRESS OUR ANGER

We can feel anger during our visit with the doctor for many reasons. We can be angry at ourselves for our failure to pursue the change we want; at the doctor, or someone else, because of our illness; or at loved ones for lack of support—or perhaps we are laboring under anger as a frequent uninvited guest in our minds, something we can't control.

When anger appears in the context of our relationship with the doctor, what can we do about it? There are two immediate options to consider: whether we should mention it at all or whether we should keep it under wraps. The present-day culture of medicine, from the biomedical roots that are firmly planted during the education of doctors and extending to the design of clinics, the personality and approach of administrators, and the lighting and design of the offices themselves make the display and acknowledgment of open emotion anathema.

Not acknowledging such a powerful emotion (anger) might be the most intuitive move, but it might not be the most productive in the long run. It could be as helpful, or more so, to find a method to convey your anger to your doctor and try to establish a line of communication concerning the issue that has elicited your anger.

How can this be done? Is it enough, or even possible, to tell the doctor you are feeling angry? I think, admittedly without strong empirical evidence to back this up, that anger pushes a huge red button in the mind of everyone privy to a conversation, and the danger is that other important elements of doctor-patient communication will go ignored after it is pressed. It might be better to talk about the anger somewhat obliquely. I am going to take the example of one patient's anger with me (suitably changing the identifiable information, of course), which she did me the favor of telling me about surprisingly explicitly, though with attention to my need for respect and order.

Ms. Denga: Doctor Berger, I really need to speak to you about something; this is very important and I am very upset.

Me: [worried] Sure, Ms. Denga, what can I help you with?

Ms. Denga: I learned from a note that was sent me that you had said that I used obscene language during the visit.

Me: Tell me why that makes you upset.

Ms. Denga: I just want to make sure that people know that I am not a person who uses obscenities with my doctor.

Me: The way I do things, is I try to record exactly what someone says during the visit—that conveys useful information to me and to other doctors.

Ms. Denga: Oh . . . as long as that's the reason. But I am upset about something else as well.

Me: You do seem angry.

Ms. Denga: Oh, no! I am not angry. I am merely upset about something else that we need to address.

Me: What is that?

Ms. Denga: At the last visit you said that you thought I had fibromyalgia. I went home and looked it up on the Internet, and they were talking a lot about chronic pain with psychiatric problems. I am not a crazy person and I won't tolerate being called a crazy person!

There is a considerable stigma attached to mental illness and its treatment. Had Ms. Denga not expressed her anger to me, I might never have known her true feelings about the subject. Many of us have been told any number of times by our doctors that we need to see this or that specialist, start taking one or the other medicine, or pursue some sort of life change. More often than not the doctor does not realize that embarking upon such a change is a huge task. No wonder then that we can get annoyed, frustrated, even furious at thoughtless assumptions about our lives, our circumstances, and what we are capable of. In short, anger can be informational and its judicious use can accelerate the process of making doctors aware of what we are thinking and feeling. (Note that I am not talking about aggressive behavior directed at doctor or patient, which no one likes and can rupture a relationship irreversibly.)

FEAR: ANTICIPATING THE UNKNOWN

Fear is another emotion that is too common in the medical encounter. I am not talking about those life and death decisions involving late-night tragedies in the emergency room or the intensive care unit. We will talk more about those in the next chapter. I am talking about the fears that, rationally or irrationally, can accompany the seemingly most innocuous of encounters. Perhaps, whenever you get dizzy, you think of your grandfather who evinced just this symptom before his stroke. Or maybe your chest pain—though the doctor has told you it has nothing to do with your heart—freezes you in your tracks every time it comes on after a quiet dinner. Fears can govern us against our wishes, but—like anger—they can also open a door onto chambers of innermost thoughts that often go uncommunicated.

Saying that you are scared is just as hard as saying you're angry. The reflexive response on the part of many doctors, when faced by someone who reports fear, is to reassure them, either that they are not in fact scared, or that they have nothing to be scared of. This reaction can trace its lineage directly to the mythical adage of the pediatrician, "This won't hurt a bit," even though many knowledgeable pediatricians don't say that anymore, knowing that it can hurt.

Many things can go wrong in medicine. No one can promise a treatment that will work 100 percent of the time, and every treatment can lead to unforeseen side effects. We all know stories about horrible things that went wrong with our relatives and friends, whether they saw a doctor or they didn't. No wonder then that many of us are scared when it comes to contemplating courses of medical treatment. Yet when today's doctors discuss the ways that people (both patients and doctors) make decisions, they often make use of the latest findings of cognitive science without considering the importance of emotions and communication.

Fear comes up differently from anger during the medical visit. Anger is elicited by states of affairs that have already occurred or are occurring right now, while fear can be mixed, agonizingly and terribly, with anticipation of things that might go wrong in the future. Since we know that things can go wrong at every step of the clinic visit—it's not just in the hospital that our safety and health can be at risk—we should anticipate that fear might be present in the exam room at every step as well, as part of the anticipation of errors or mere dread of the unknown.

Take the very start of the visit, where we are discussing our history, both personal and familial, with the doctor. We all have relatives who have had terrible health problems, and few of us can help hoping and wishing that we never experience what the person who had the painful disease or the premature death did. Such hopes and premonitions can be helpful in some cases, motivating us to behavioral change. [8]

Health economists talk about the "gamble" that can be simulated to help us figure out which alternative would be more palatable in the context of medical decision making. For example, would you take such-and-such a medication if there were, say, a 25 percent chance you would have to be on dialysis for the rest of your life after taking it? Such grim trade-offs are commonplace in the world of statisticians who try to estimate our health preferences—without really ever having met us. [9]

Fear is not easily addressed by the paradigm of cause, treatment, and improvement that many doctors gravitate to. There is some evidence that a brief session of reassurance can reduce fear. [10] But I have seen too many doctors who seem to be expert in false reassurance, saying the wrong thing at the wrong time. I assume I have done so as well. If you are reassured in the wrong way, the worries you have had might not be quieted, while things you weren't even worrying about previously might come to the fore.

The only way to address fear, in some cases, might not be to say, falsely, "It will be all right," according to some doctors' misguided instinct, or to discuss statistics that the concern is overblown, but to rely on us, the patients, to address the concern in some concrete way with the doctor. Is there a test that has few downsides that can provide concrete data to reassure? Would there be signs of the terrible outcome you worry about that you should be on the watch for?

To take one example, I recently saw a woman in her forties with a history of a benign mass that had previously been removed from one side of her neck. She came to see me worrying about a sensation of fullness in the other side of her neck. I examined her, and it really didn't seem as though there was anything there.

The question was, at this point, what to do about it. If you are thinking I performed some magic of doctor-patient communication at this moment, you are mistaken. I was groping in the dark like so many doctors are, just trying to find the right thing to say that would not make a bad impression. *Primum non nocere*—first do no harm, as the founder of the doctor's guild put it. "I'm not sure it's . . . dangerous," I said gingerly after examining the patient and indeed finding nothing in the neck worth the chilling name "mass." "But we could take a picture."

"What kind of picture?" she asked, interested but not yet convinced. "One option is a CT scan, but that would open you up to the risk of radiation. Instead, maybe we can consider an ultrasound. It would give some indication of whether there is, in fact, anything there." She agreed to that, mollified if not completely free of concerns. Note that I did not say, "it's nothing," on the one hand, or offer, on the other hand, something on the other end of the testing or imaging spectrum, such as an MRI of the neck, say, or a referral to an endocrinologist. Not that I have anything against such modalities or strategies per se. But in a situation where I was pretty sure there was no problem in her neck, I wanted to err on the side of doing as little as possible and still reassure her.

The end of the story isn't so surprising—there wasn't any mass found by the ultrasound after all. The results came back, and I told her about them. I don't know if she was reassured, but it was at least a response to her concerns.

The more difficult case, obviously, is when you are scared because of something terrible that has been diagnosed or that you think is about to happen. We will talk about such situations in the next chapter.

OUR APPROACH TO SADNESS

After anger and fear, the next most common emotion in the doctor-patient visit, at least according to my experience, is sadness. Sadness comes in many levels. There is a whole spectrum extending from a down mood, on the one hand, to full-blown severe clinical depression on the other.

The approach to sadness should vary with its place along the emotional spectrum. Mild sadness—having a bad day—can be addressed by talking it through or by the tincture of time. The harder question is what to do about more severe sadness—what we call depression.

I am aware that it is frowned upon in many circles to equate sadness, a common emotion, to depression, a clinical condition. One is a part of life with its ups and downs, the other is a medical problem that can be successfully treated with medication or psychotherapy.

Or is that last part really true? Is depression, the clinical syndrome, really clearly distinguishable from garden-variety sadness? Is the necessity of and susceptibility to treatment with medication and therapy really clear?

As with so many other items of medical orthodoxy, the answer is not all that clear. Realizing the difficulty of this problem can also help us all understand how gingerly we need to approach the medical treatment of what, in many cases, might be everyday emotions. Respect for the place of emotions in the doctor-patient encounter also means that we all should know when to step aside and let the emotions take their course.

While just a few years ago it seemed to many physicians that there was a consensus regarding the treatment of depression—that for even moderate depression, pharmacotherapy was at least equal in effectiveness to psychotherapy—now there is more and more evidence that the studies of medications for the treatment of depression are marred by bias.[11] For example, differences reported as significant from a statistical point of view are not clinically significant at all, patients are not randomly selected to receive treatment, and so on. Not only that, these deficiencies have been underreported, or glossed over, in the literature on the treatment of depression. Doctors might have been lulled into overprescribing depression medications—not out of any sinister motives on their part, but because of their wish to help patients—and also, unfortunately, pushed by the big and often deleterious influence of large pharmaceutical companies.

So depression is not something that should automatically be treated with medication. There is a spectrum. The same can be said of anger and anxiety—they are not always clinical syndromes, but can be understood according to a different model. According to the disease model, symptoms arise from pathology—something is broken, and this leads to what can be called depression or anxiety. But according to a behavioral model, these symptoms can be adaptive responses to outside stressors.

We need to be careful in the visit, as doctors and patients, not to attribute emotional responses to personality faults or undiscovered psychopathology. Emotions can be, first and foremost, responses, and should be recognized as such.[12]

I have talked about emotion during the doctor-patient encounter, and how it might be present at many parts of the visit. Emotions are important because they show us a face of health care that is different from some trends that are now fashionable. These days there is quite an emphasis placed on decision making and making sure that we all share in the decision-making process to the extent of our wishes and abilities. In fact, some people go so far as to say that the point of the medical encounter from the patient's point of view should be such shared decision making.[13]

I disagree with this assessment. As we discussed in chapter 1, the medical interview has several functions, including building rapport between doctor and patient, gathering information, and education—on both sides. Decision making can be a part of a medical visit, but not necessarily. To limit health care to decisions betrays a bias from the cognitive sciences, which are undeniably powerful and of interest, and are undergoing something of a spike in popularity. Much of medical errors and the imperfections of our health care system are placed at the feet of cognitive biases and barriers.

However, there are plenty of visits in which no decision is made. Events are discussed, support is provided, courses of action are talked about, but nothing is decided. Sometimes it is enough to talk through things and discuss experiences. Visits can also be important tools in addressing areas in our lives that we are nervous about bringing up with the doctor, areas we will discuss in the next chapter.

Chapter Eleven

How to Talk to the Doctor About What Makes You Nervous, Embarrassed, or Grossed Out

I was seeing a patient, whose identity I have obviously concealed for the purposes of this story to respect her confidentiality. She was in her fifties, a professional woman, and very educated, independent, and articulate, not at all the sort of person whom you would think is often caught like a deer in the headlights. She had called my office asking for an acute visit; in other words, she had an important matter she wanted to discuss.

She seemed her normal self when she sat down, polished and in control. "Doctor, I have a problem," she began.

"Yes?" I responded, listening.

"It's a problem down there," she said significantly, and looked at me directly. I had no idea what she was talking about.

"Down there?" I said.

"Yes, you know."

"No," I said. "I don't. Is it a problem urinating?"

No, she said, it wasn't that.

"Do you have burning or discharge from your vagina?"

Not that either. She denied abdominal pain, constipation, diarrhea, blood in her stool, or any change in her bowel movement habits.

After going through a laundry list of questions, I asked her about something else, a more sensitive topic and something that, to be honest, the two of us had never before addressed in a visit. "Tell me about your sexual activity," I offered. "Are you having any problems there?" "Yes," she said, and looked relieved. "Yes, I am. That's what I meant."

I remember us both laughing at that time. It was an awkward moment—it had taken us no little back-and-forth to get to the relatively simple matter, medically speaking, of pain during sex.

There were several reasons it took us too long to get to that point. First is the most obvious reason. I'm a man, she's a woman, and she would be more likely to divulge such concerns to a female doctor.[1] How many women feel uncomfortable bringing up their complaints to their primary care doctor because that doctor is a man? However, even if we take gender discordance into account, there are other reasons that apply here.

One overarching truth explains many of these reasons quite simply. The encounter with the doctor hinges on truths that can make us worried, scared, disgusted, or embarrassed—occasionally all at the same time. In one visit, we might have to talk about our urine, bowel movements, sexual function, pain, fear of losing our mind, and our financial and emotional worries—and this doesn't even include the end we all have in common, death.

We can sweep these things under the rug, which might make for less awkward visits. But then who are we going to talk about these matters with? How can we base the visit on a productive relationship if we are leaving our most serious and personal issues on the other side of the office door?

Just as in the previous chapter I talked about the emotions that are difficult to deal with during the encounter with the doctor, in this chapter I will talk about the issues that hardly anyone finds easy to talk about, whether because they are intimate physiological processes or because they expose our frailties and imperfections.

GENERAL STRATEGIES TO DISCUSS THINGS THAT MAKE YOU UNCOMFORTABLE

First, let's discuss several general strategies that can be applied to many such topics. Any of these sensitive matters, whether it's sex, farting, or your bowels, can be "medicalized," or discussed in technical language. In the study I conducted about the ways in which patients expressed the reasons for their admission to the hospital,[2] many patients used diagnostic language to explain the reason for their admission, while I had hypothesized beforehand that people would be more likely to talk about their problems in terms of their symptoms—how they feel. People *can* think in "medical terms" (i.e., using diagnostic terminology) more often, and more in keeping with the way doctors use them, than we give ourselves credit for.

I am not saying that you need to become a walking medical encyclopedia, or open up a medical website any time you have a problem urinating or a sexual issue. But, on occasion, using professional, specific language can make a difference in how others perceive your problems.

The second general strategy is to recognize that you are not the first person to be embarrassed about your bodily functions. While many people have no problem, it seems, and discuss their every movement via social media, many others of us are not that way and get nervous about disclosing our innermost workings, even to a doctor. One suggestion is to tell the doctor frankly about our discomfort.

There are also strategies appropriate to each area which might make these sensitive topics a little less sensitive, or at least fit them into the context of the healthy relationship.

BOWELS AND OTHER PARTS

Every stage of life brings its particular bowel changes, workings, and dysfunctions—starting from bowel training of toddlers, to the effects of diet changes or alcohol use, to the bowel problems that come about with middle or old age.

One common complaint that is uncommonly revealed in the later decades of life is fecal incontinence, losing stool. Who wants to talk about that? The scientific literature suggests, however, that many doctors do not even ask about it. So if you are suffering from it, and don't figure out a way to bring it up, your doctor might never think to mention it. Perhaps doctors themselves are also, in these areas, susceptible to the same reflexive attitudes of disgust that people everywhere are.[3]

Urine incontinence is another common issue, and another problem that many people are too self-conscious to bring up. Being able to discuss this with the doctor, however, might initiate a discussion about options for treatment. If you and your doctor do not communicate about how often you lose urine, what the things are that set it off, what treatments you have tried, and what steps you might be willing to take in the future, you might be missing an opportunity to improve your symptoms.

Even trickier than bowel problems is the discussion of urinary symptoms, in part because remedies for urinary symptoms are widely advertised, albeit of mixed effectiveness. So you have to be clear, with yourself and with the doctor, about how long your symptoms have lasted, how disruptive they are, and whether you would like to embark on treatments for them.

SEX

I admit that I, myself, as a doctor and a patient, find it uncomfortable to discuss sex. While bowel and bladder function is difficult enough, discussion of sexual practices is still often glossed over or omitted by the physician.[4] Perhaps the doctor assumes that the person in front of them is too old to have sex, too buttoned-up to have unsafe sex, or too different from the doctor (lesbian, gay, or transgender) for the doctor to think about the patient's sexual health.

Yes, the doctor should ask about urine and bowel movements at every visit, and sex should be discussed at every regular visit, too. It's not just that things can go wrong in the bedroom—from sexual dysfunction to unsafe sex to sexually transmitted infection—but sex can be a bellwether, an indication of how things are going in our lives in general. And, since about a third to a half of everyone who sees the doctor for the first time has some sort of problem with sexual function,[5] it behooves doctors to ask.

There are a number of guides that tell doctors how to take a complete history of sex. It's useful for you to understand these questions so that you can be prepared—and noticing your doctor's approach to the sexual history can be a window onto their ability to conduct the interview in a way that allows for conversation.

As in other parts of the medical interview, it is suggested that doctors should start out "open-ended," asking general questions first before honing in on the specific complaints we bring to the visit. However, we have to be careful in our visit with the doctor not to gloss over areas that we might be uncomfortable talking about. If we plan to go to the doctor to talk about some specific area of sexual concern, and we respond vaguely, with generalities, we might lead ourselves down the wrong path.

If we do bring up sexual problems when talking to the doctor, it's our job in the conversation to get specific about the problem. Is it that we lack desire or that we have a physiological problem? Do we have pain with intercourse? Do we have a problem maintaining erections or with orgasm?

Some of the most sensitive issues have to do with our sexual partners— and these are the issues that doctors often have the most problems asking about. That is, whether we are having sex with men, women, or both; if we are having unsafe sex, with multiple partners; whether we are using protection; and what kind of sex we are having. Many people have recourse to columnists and informal advice givers because they are uncomfortable bringing up these issues with their doctors. Sex involves taboos, but if we are clear and specific about our symptoms, we might be able to talk about more with our doctor than we expect.

HOW WE DIE—AND (DON'T) TALK ABOUT DEATH

The most sensitive issue of all in our medical lives is how our lives end. The fact that Americans from many walks of life are unnaturally separated from a practical consideration of their future death has been amply discussed.[6] And there are strategies that have been suggested to make people communicate.

The problem is that these strategies amount to protocols that prompt doctor or patient to check in on specific areas of end-of-life care. The Physician Orders for Life Sustaining Treatment,[7] for example, is a form that a doctor can fill out in conversation with you about your preferences regarding end-of-life treatments—whether you might prefer not to get intravenous fluids, for example, or whether you would want to avoid measures to restart your heart after it stops, or have a breathing tube put down your throat in case of respiratory distress.

Similarly, there are an increasing number of initiatives that encourage us to make plans for our end-of-life care. The centerpiece of these plans is usually the living will, directions to our surrogates as to our wishes when we can no longer make medical decisions.

There are at least two kinds of problems with these directions we leave in case we are no longer *compos mentis*. First, we often change our decisions with time, especially decisions dependent on circumstances, our emotions, and our own relationships to family and friends. Second, most of us have little first-hand knowledge about the end of life, the medical options that are available, and to what extent they help.[8]

This means that if we are unavailable to decide about such matters or cognitively weakened due to disease, our loved ones or whomever we have chosen are left to make decisions that we are not able to make. They are left squeezed from all sides: they feel terrible making decisions that they feel unequipped to make, thinking that if they only knew what we wanted, they might have an easier time of it and be able to represent our final wishes more authentically.[9]

As a result, certain bioethicists, most notably Daniel Sulmasy of the University of Chicago, have promoted a different route to helping our surrogates make end-of-life decisions: engage them, and us, in discussions, based on narrative, of what we find important in life.[10] Such narratives represent our basic values, and it is those values that surrogates can faithfully communicate, even if they are lost in the minutiae of whether we would want a breathing tube.

Such a discussion would theoretically go something like the following, assuming that a relative of ours was in the hospital very ill, unable for whatever reason to make a decision about his health.

Doctor: I wanted to ask you about your grandfather, and what kind of person he is. What sorts of things does he find important?

You: What do you mean, find important? He likes walking in the woods, fishing, spending time with his grandchildren, watching football on TV . . .

Doctor: Have there ever been any situations where a relative, or someone you were close to, had to make decisions about the end of their life and what interventions they wanted to pursue?

[you look blank]

Doctor: What I mean is, have you ever had a relative in a similar situation?

You: Oh, yes, my mother was in the intensive care unit for weeks. We tried to do everything. She was on all sorts of machines. And I know that . . . I'm not sure they did anything for her. Everyone thought we should take her off them. But I thought it was really doing something for her.

Doctor: And what did your father think about all this?

You: I'm not sure. I think we talked about it, but I think he was pretty conflicted.

You see the problem. There are decisions to be made that affect how people die—people whom you love very much. You might need to act in someone's stead, or appoint someone to act at a time when you can no longer do so. A previous generation's advice was to give particular directions, but it turns out that many people don't understand what these directions mean, either because they are not familiar with the terminology or because it's difficult to predict our wishes ahead of time, let alone the wishes of other people.

The alternative, to figure out someone's end of life wishes through a discussion of the priorities that were evident in their life, is a great idea but difficult in practice. How often can we point to someone's life and say that it was lived according to something more than vague principles? Can you think of your own explicitly formed life philosophies, particularly around an issue as sensitive as the end of your life? Even more, can you divine your relative's desires through your interactions with her, even if these interactions are not particularly philosophical or thought through?

I don't have a perfect answer to this conundrum. There is no solution to the matter of discussing one's end of life preferences that would satisfy all parties: sick people, their relatives, and their doctors. Instead of protocols and scripts, the conversation about end-of-life preferences might better be founded on the basis of a relationship.

THE DOCTOR-PATIENT RELATIONSHIP AND END-OF-LIFE CARE: A STORY

I was seeing a patient once in the clinic and I got an urgent page. Surprised and not a little annoyed, I excused myself and went into another room. An ICU nurse was trying to reach me, which confused me somewhat. Although doctors often fail to tell another doctor when their patient is in the hospital, I usually find that my colleagues in Johns Hopkins do inform me: at the very least, when my patient is in the intensive care unit. Yet, I had no recollection of a patient of mine ending up there recently.

But there was a patient of mine in the intensive care unit, as it turned out. The nurse told me that Mr. Gonzalez (whose name I have changed) had been there a week with sepsis, widespread infection that was life threatening. The source had been traced to his colon: there was an abscess in it, and the surgeons were proposing to take it out as a practicable, if not a simple or risk free, way of getting rid of the infection, thus the sepsis—and thus saving the patient's life. All good intentions.

I hadn't seen Mr. Gonzalez in two and a half years, nearly as long as I had been at Hopkins at that point. We had seen each other a grand total of twice in the clinic. I had to look up the medical record to even remind myself who he was. We had not had a meaningful conversation, or so I thought.

However, as the team in the intensive care unit told me, when the family discovered that a fateful decision lay in front of them, and their Mr. Gonzalez was not able to make the decision for himself, they asked for the doctor he had only met twice before. They had never heard of me, but they tracked me down.

One of the surgical nurse practitioners was the one who had paged me. She had called me from the conference room, where she and Mr. Gonzalez's family were meeting with the rest of the treatment team. "When does this decision have to be made?" I asked her. "Basically within a couple of hours—is it okay if I put the family on the phone?"

It was Mr. Gonzalez's wife who finally talked to me after the phone was passed a bit from hand to hand among the family members. Mrs. Gonzalez and I had met during one of those uneventful clinic visits, although I didn't remember meeting her. She said, "The surgeons tell us that they need to do a procedure to remove some of his infected intestine."

"Yes," I said, "but I'm afraid I don't have any more exact information than that. They are the experts as far as this procedure goes."

"I understand," she said. "But I wanted to know what you would do in this situation."

"It depends on what you think is important," I said carefully. "The procedure might save his life, but he could be forever changed afterwards; he could have brain or organ damage that would make him unable to do some of the activities he could do before."

"So you think we should do it?" she asked.

I gnashed my teeth quietly. What I wanted least to do was to tell this family—who I didn't really know—what to do!

But I told them: "It seems like Mr. Gonzalez is quite seriously ill, and the surgeons think they can do something that can help him. It really depends on balancing priorities—if you want to make sure Mr. Gonzalez has a chance at life, the operation might be something to choose. As long as . . . " (here I started speaking faster, because I felt that the family member was about to get off the phone) ". . . you realize that his life might be very different after the operation. That's something you should take into account."

The family chose to have the operation. Mr. Gonzalez survived and actually did quite well, but for one reason or another I have not seen him or his family since. It was as if the relationship was something for them to hold onto in the moment, even if, after the threat of death, they realized they didn't need it anymore.

Mr. Gonzalez had left precious little written instruction, like many of us, about what he wanted at the end of his life. So what does this story of mine tell us about how we should prepare ourselves and our families for such a situation?

We see that trying to leave written directions foreseeing such a situation is part of the solution, but not all of it, because these directions might not reflect current reality, and might be ignored by the doctors on the scene. Often the treating physicians do not know where these documents are kept and might be at a loss when it comes to interpreting them, even if they can be found at the right moment. Appointing surrogates to make decisions on your behalf, or on your family member's behalf, is another part of the solution, but not every family member wants to be put in that position. The experience may be stressful, even life changing and traumatic. Furthermore, the decision the surrogate eventually makes might not reflect the wishes of the person they are making the decision for.

If written directions and surrogates have their downsides, then relying on what the person found important in their life also has its weaknesses: for what, at bottom, can we understand about a fellow human being's deepest wants and desires unless we know them well over an extended period of time? Family members are not necessarily always in touch with each other over a number of years, and the person we are talking about might have changed in the meantime. The religious young man we knew and loved might have morphed into a militant atheist. The acolyte of medical technology, struck by the dehumanized last days of her grandmother, might decide she no longer believes in the benefit of intensive interventions in the ICU.

Faced with the imperfections of nearly every approach in our health care system to making the last days of our lives more reflective of what we actually want, the Gonzalez family got in touch with the primary care physician Mr. Gonzalez had seen exactly twice. Not everyone can have recourse to such a relationship, but it is a possible alternative among those I have already mentioned.

What can the relationship bring to the discussion of end-of-life care, apart from the desperate reaching for a familiar name that impelled the Gonzalez family to seek me out? There is knowledge of the personality and priorities from a family member; there is comfort with the end-of-life situation, something that spooks many laypeople; and there is the ability to be in contact with many sources of medical information at once.

I am not saying that doctors should take the place of the patients themselves or of their designated surrogates or family members. But it is interesting to me that in the various protocols, strategies, and interventions revolving around our discussions of end-of-life care, few of them make use of the precious resource, relationship, that I have spent much of this book talking about. There are serious situations in life where we ask advice of someone who knows us well. What better person, in the medical context, than our doctors, if we have a relationship and they have the knowledge to help us through?

MENTAL HEALTH AND THE DOCTOR-PATIENT RELATIONSHIP

I'll finish this chapter with a sensitive issue that is even less addressed, by some doctors, than our plans for the end of life: our mental health. While we all die, and some of us are comfortable talking about it, discussions about our mental health are still considerably stigmatized, making it an issue of great discomfort and nervousness for many of us.

Mental health problems are common, with the prevalence of depression in the general population around 10 percent. This is not as high as diabetes or high blood pressure but certainly common enough so that one doctor, in a usual clinic day of seeing about twenty or thirty patients, should see at least one person with depression. General anxiety disorder is more or less as common.

Add to these disorders all the different mental health problems that are slightly less common—panic disorder, bipolar disorder, adjustment disorder, dysthymia (short-term depressed mood)—and one begins to see that most people in a given day of a doctor's clinic might have some sort of mental health problem.

There are also challenges we face in mental health that cannot be diagnosed through the psychiatrists' *Diagnostic and Statistical Manual.* The issues we are struggling with, from our childhood, home life, work stressors, or causes of worry and sadness, might not meet diagnostic criteria. Nevertheless, mental health can significantly affect physical health. Even the garden-variety doctor should be prepared to help such people during a visit, and to think about the interaction between physical and mental problems.

Despite these facts, and the widespread nature of mental health problems, many of us are still loath to bring them up when we see our doctor. There are several obvious reasons for this. There is a stigma: we don't want to be thought of as "crazy," or that our symptoms are "all in our head."

Even though we expect our doctors to be able to connect physical and mental symptoms, and to be comfortable with how the two interact, such an appreciation is not regularly conveyed in the current curricula of medical schools. According to the Oslerian model of the ideal physician, the true medical professional puts his or her emotions aside. There is empathy, yes, but it is of the distant clinical variety, not the sensitivity to the entire emotional field that can exist as part of a doctor-patient encounter. Thus, doctors might not be trained to pick up the nervousness with which we approach discussions of our mental health.

Some doctors, in other words, might be as uncomfortable as we are in talking about depression, anxiety, bipolar disorder, and substance abuse, or talking about the thought that symptoms are getting control of us, and that our body is rebelling against the brain.

Two strategies can help get you on the same page as your doctor when it comes to discussing your psychological health.

First, connect the psychological to the physiological. I am not the first to mention that symptoms of mind and body are connected. Nevertheless, mind-body medicine has a bad name in certain quarters—it has a whiff of the homeopathic or the granola, and even the academic, federally funded variety of alternative and complementary medicine does not have the support of a considerable body of scientific evidence, or respect from many doctors.

But if you can approach the doctor with this connection, and put on the table that you think some of your symptoms are affected by your mental state, you can start the conversation off in the right direction. Because the doctor, once she has ruled out any dangerous causes of your problem, should want to improve matters just like you.

Second, present the connection between your mental state, the stressors in your life, and your physical state as a *fait accompli* with a symptom diary. A symptom diary is an opportunity for you to be exact with your own recollections for your own and your doctor's use. The trick with a symptom diary, however, is that it is up to you to include the categories that you think might be affecting your symptoms. If you think that your stomach pains are worsened by your mood—or, contrariwise, have nothing to do with any mind-body connection—then that should be something that the categories of your symptom diary should allow you to record.

The advice I have given thus far is more appropriate for those who are facing psychiatric or psychological conditions of moderate severity. Quite a different tack is needed, obviously, if you are suffering from a severe psychiatric disorder. Reading this book is probably not the first step you are taking to treat your symptoms, I hope.

There are cases, however, where your primary physician might not be keen on treating your mental health condition, and you do not have a mental health provider that you trust. In that case, you might have to make your own judgment about the risks and benefits and, perhaps, approach your regular doctor with an unconventional suggestion: that you and he work on your mental health treatment together. If you and your doctor can't do it, and you can't find a psychiatrist who fills the bill, who else can?

WHEN THE DOCTOR IS NERVOUS: HOW TO HELP YOU AND YOUR DOCTOR BE MORE COMFORTABLE WITH SENSITIVE TOPICS

The readiness of doctors to talk about these sensitive topics—urine, bowel movements, sex, and mental health—is still incomplete. Many of them are still uncomfortable doing so. We can change this lack of comfort only so much. We need to realize the reasons that underlie this nervousness, and try to address them in a systematic way.

In medical school and residency, training in communication with patients used to be thin on the ground. More and more, such training is recognized as important. Indeed, modules on doctor-patient communication have been added to the curricula of many medical schools. In many places, simulated patients are the core of these curricula, putting students and residents through their paces as they speak to actors expertly trained in acting like real sick people.[11] Training students and residents is an exercise in balancing priorities. If you are to choose certain medical conditions that should form the background of communication or relationship training for students of residents, it stands to reason that the most common medical conditions chosen would be diabetes, heart disease, and high blood pressure, which do not necessarily encompass the emotionally sensitive issues that we have discussed in this chapter.

Thus a vicious cycle is created. Since these sensitive issues are not often brought up, medical students and residents do not find themselves comfortable discussing them with patients. The students and residents are trained in and help implement curricula for those who come after them—curricula that do not include teaching students or residents how to talk to patients about these issues. And so these unaddressed matters go on, important to us but underaddressed in medical visits.

When medical schools and the doctors who come out of them are not sufficiently trained in this or any other area, sometimes it behooves us and our communities as a whole to step up and make change. In the coming chapter we will talk about how to do that.

Chapter Twelve

Making Healthy Communities with Healthy Communication

Our visit with the doctor lasts fifteen minutes by the clock, but we live our lives every single moment, bearing the burden of disease or glimpsing the far-off horizon of health. The principles I have discussed can support our health even outside of the doctor's office. We need to be emotionally and intellectually ready. We must have our agenda in hand. And we can, at that moment, acknowledge and make use of emotions to help us maintain health and conquer disease through motivation.

Doctors too have come to realize that the office encounter is only the tip of the iceberg. Outside the walls of the clinic, the struggle between health and illness is going on all the time. The health of individuals is bound up with the health of the community. Physicians have usually seen their work as separate from that of public health professionals: doctors treat, public health workers prevent. Physicians counsel us about our options, guiding us to a decision; public health workers make it their business to legislate good health behaviors.

This dichotomy is exaggerated, though the tension between the two professions is real. Luckily enough, each one of us can attempt to bridge these two different worlds. We do this through taking our decision-making capacities and using them for the health of our communities.

This chapter will discuss health conditions in which ordinary people have made a difference in their health environments, using the principles of communication that I have outlined in previous chapters.

THE HEALTHY INDIVIDUAL, THE HEALTH OF THE COMMUNITY

Before I discuss the health conditions, however, we should have in mind the ideal relationship of individual and community. We are accustomed to seeing ourselves as part of a greater good, in terms of politics, since we share in a common self-definition as Americans, or economics, since we are part of a common market. But what is the common market of our health? If it is true that a butterfly flapping its wings in Brazil can bring about a tornado in China, can the actions of one person influence the health of an entire society?

There are some obvious examples of the relationship between individual and community and its impact on health. The widespread effectiveness of vaccines depends upon herd immunity. If individuals find it inadvisable to be vaccinated, then the vaccine itself will be less effective. Similarly, people's individual behaviors can affect the prevalence of sexually transmitted infections.

What about for chronic, not infectious conditions? Even if they are not passed from person to person by infectious agents, many health conditions are influenced by the society that the individual is a part of.[1]

The smallest relevant scale in which one person can affect the health of others is in the family unit. Outside the family a person is part of a culture. A culture has particular ways of thinking about relationships between behavior and health, called explanatory models (EMs) in the scientific literature. These EMs can play an important role in the community's understanding of its own health, as a recent research article shows; and while the article did not explicitly examine the change that one individual can make in a community's "health culture," it provides some tantalizing hints.

The study, published in the *Journal of General Internal Medicine*,[2] examined how health messages tailored to a particular minority group, Americans of Southeast Asian descent, are received by that group. Knowing that Southeast Asians are the second fastest growing ethnic group in the United States, with rates of heart disease higher than other ethnic groups, the researchers decided to target Southeast Asians with a video encouraging screening for, and modification of risk factors associated with, heart disease. They tried to incorporate the ways in which Southeast Asians view heart disease according to their explanatory models.

However, the video was not received in the way researchers expected. Some members of the target audience who saw it objected to the forthright language about the risk of heart disease in Southeast Asians, characterizing it as a "bold attack." These people preferred instead to hear about the ways the community had made, and could continue to make, progress in combating heart disease. As a result, the video was modified.

The study does not measure the success of the video in recruiting Southeast Asians to help reduce their community's risk of heart disease. But the connection between the individual, the community, and the explanatory model is something that can apply to everyone, as can the necessity of modifying the explanatory model when it does not fit a particular community.

WAYS TO UNDERSTANDING HEALTH: OUR EXPLANATORY MODELS AND OUR DOCTORS' APPROACH TO MEDICINE

The explanatory model is a theoretical construct to understand a community's approach to disease. While the orthodox medical understanding is that turbulent blood flow, extra work by the heart, or greater than normal constriction in the blood vessel walls causes elevated blood pressure, many people throughout the world have different ways to talk about the causes of high blood pressure. Stress, as I mentioned above, is a common candidate, but so are headaches, "bad blood," and other factors. And each of these factors has to lead in certain ways to high blood pressure for the connection to make sense.

I am not going to take off my white doctor's coat and tear my diploma off the wall. I believe in medical explanations more than folk explanations. But the explanatory model is something that cannot be abandoned so easily. Each of us has our own health beliefs which impact how we behave. Our actions, in turn, affect those around us, and so on in a ripple effect

Our layperson beliefs about health and wellness, not hewing to chapter and verse of medical science but not ignoring it either, can spread little by little into the explanatory models of our friends, partners, and relations, for the health of all of us.

A controversial example of this line of thinking is vaccines. The great majority of scientists know that vaccines prevent infections, sometimes deadly infections, in children. But the scientific literature, is more complicated than that, as in so many other examples. A recent meta-analysis (statistical combination of studies) of the effectiveness of the flu vaccine, using the recently available, highly sensitive tests for the influenza virus, found that "Influenza vaccines can provide moderate protection against virologically confirmed influenza, but such protection is greatly reduced or absent in some seasons."[3] As I read these words as a doctor, my heart sank as I thought of all my patients who would grimace when I recommended this year's flu vaccine. I couldn't imagine that calling it "moderately" effective would make them, or me, any more enthusiastic to get the shot.

Understandably, Arthur Caplan, a well-known bioethicist formerly at the University of Pennsylvania and now at New York University Medical Center, where I was a resident, squawked at this finding and called publishing it irresponsible. If the meta-analysis was publicized, and picked up by the media, it could convince the public that the flu vaccine did not work at all. This matters because herd immunity, in which a large group of people undergo immunization, reducing the transmission of the virus, is essential to reduce the spread of an infectious agent.[4]

What is the everyday person supposed to think if the scientific literature does not yet "prove" the effectiveness of a vaccine that many doctors take to be a given? There are always gaps between the ways in which doctors and researchers understand medical information and the way that the public approaches it. Someone told me the other day that, while the influenza vaccine might work on groups of people, there are certain people it just doesn't work for—like him; could I write him a letter confirming this?

I propose a compromise between rigorous scientific research and the naïve understanding of the public. Taking the example of vaccines, it is undeniable that any shot can be associated with adverse effects (perhaps those go underemphasized in the push to vaccinate every last patient). By the same token, however, the truth that vaccines prevent the flu has become widely accepted among certain communities, even if we cannot always explain the exact mechanisms of the protection.

This is not true of every community, however—differences in vaccination rates vary among subpopulations.[5] In other words, among some groups of people, the vaccine is less popular. This is where things get tricky. Identifying subgroups among patients has been done for good and for ill, and the issue of health-care disparities, differences in health care quality or behavior between subgroups, is a very sensitive one. For example, African Americans have been specially exploited by doctors and researchers,[6] so it is no surprise that the residual mistrust of medicine among African Americans is not insignificant.[7]

If one is in that community and feels that the flu vaccine works, what is the best way for that person to go about influencing others without being a person no one wants to talk to, a self-righteous annoyance? You can take it upon yourself to spread healthy messages without driving away other people. We can learn what not to do from advertising campaigns that might in fact get on the nerves of many of us: awareness-raising messages for issues like breast cancer that don't need a lot of awareness raised, since research and clinical care for the disease is relatively well supported. There are issues that can reach awareness saturation with the public and for which screening might currently be overpromoted.[8]

Some methods to improve your group's use of health services might be relatively straightforward. If your friends or family are skeptical about vaccinations, you can talk about your experience or the evidence you have read. If there are unhealthy behaviors prevalent in your community, you might have influence to help decrease them.

SAVING LIVES IN YOUR COMMUNITY: EMPOWERING PEOPLE TO CHANGE THEMSELVES

For some health conditions, however, the best way to address disparities, differences in treatment or outcome among different patient groups, is unclear—and the condition might be serious and deadly. In a recent article in the *New England Journal of Medicine*, researchers compared neighborhoods according to their rates of bystander cardiopulmonary resuscitation (CPR).[9] How often did everyday people standing on the street, who were not necessarily medical professionals, resuscitate someone whose heart or breathing had stopped?

It is important to interpret the results carefully. Neighborhoods that were majority African American had lower rates of bystander resuscitation compared to high-income majority white neighborhoods; compared to wealthier white neighborhoods, the rate of CPR was also lower in low-income black neighborhoods, high-income black neighborhoods, and low-income white neighborhoods. High-income integrated neighborhoods had rates of bystander CPR comparable to high-income white neighborhoods.

Why is this? First, perhaps the result isn't accurate. In many cases an interesting and publicized scientific result is a false positive, or built on mistaken assumptions. Another possibility is that the results have nothing to do with racial or ethnic categories per se, but with socioeconomic categories. There is something about disadvantaged groups of people that makes them less likely or less able to resuscitate as bystanders. Yes, low-income black neighborhoods and high-income black neighborhoods were both less likely to resuscitate than those in high-income white neighborhoods, but it could be that the income measurements of the study do not represent the full measure of the disadvantage in being a member of a minority group in the United States.

Why might one group, however defined, start CPR less than another group? Perhaps the circumstances of their community make it difficult or impossible, or maybe the members of the community lack motivation to participate. CPR, though life saving, is stressful and requires self-activation. Can we change this lack through our actions as individuals? Maybe in this case influencing the health behavior of the community around us is asking too much of us. Sometimes it's as much as we can do to change ourselves. Rather than trying to change our community, sometimes we can try to empower our community—our neighbors, friends and relatives—to change itself.

The first step is finding out what the community's priorities are. This is not always so simple. How does a community identify what it finds important? Or, to take a step back, what is the definition of a community? Saying that individuals can influence a community assumes that we can easily define who is a member of the group, or who is in or out. Perhaps you are different from the people around you, and it's all you can do just to take care of yourself. Or perhaps the group you are in has a history of negative experiences with the health-care system and, as a result, is suspicious of doctors and hospitals.

If you are part of a group that does not trust doctors or hospitals, but you are seeing benefits from a relationship with a primary care provider, you might be able to make a difference to your community by letting members know about the benefits you see from that relationship: not just by recommending this particular doctor but by talking up visiting a doctor as a resource in itself.

If you have a primary care doctor but not one you can trust, it is not always possible to go and choose a new one. But you can try to alert your doctor to the suspicions that you feel. I have a patient, I'll call her Ms. Miller, who is an African American woman in her seventies. "Doctor, I wonder if you really like me," she said, while she was sitting on the exam table and I was working on some prescription refills for her on the computer. I wasn't sure I had heard right. "Of course I like you!" I said. "I like all my patients." This of course is not exactly true, no one likes everyone, but I try to like them all well enough. After all, the doctor is supposed to have "unconditional positive regard" that enables him to build a good working relationship with the patient. "We have different skin colors," she said sort of mournfully. "Are there doctors who treat you differently because of your race?" I said. I was being somewhat disingenuous, as I knew that there is ample evidence for disparities in treatment due to different behaviors of doctors based on the race of their patients; we can straightforwardly call it racism. "Yes," she said, "and my friends and family think so too."

I tried telling her that even though we had many differences between us, I try and treat all my patients the same. But then I thought, is that really the case?

PURSUING HEALTH DIFFERENTLY IN THE CONTEXT OF YOUR COMMUNITY

Doctors do treat different groups of people differently, and every person who sees a doctor figures that out right away. But perhaps, on occasion, and excepting the invidious influence of racism, we need to be treated differently in order to make an impact on the health of our community. We can return to the example of vaccinations to make this point.

Not everyone reading these words is going to get the flu shot. There are many people who find the vaccinations unpleasant, scary, or dangerous, so I won't be able to convince them that it's something they should have if they have been avoiding it for years.

However, whichever way you tend, there should be a discussion taking place among you, your friends and neighbors, and your community at large about how you see the flu vaccine in your lives. If you think it is bad for you, a position I disagree with, you should discuss that with the people closest to you and figure out another way to protect yourself against influenza. If you think the vaccine is effective, the position I hold, then you should try to have an effect within your community to increase the proportion of people who are vaccinated.

EMPOWERING THE HEALTH OF YOUR COMMUNITY

In essence, what we are talking about is providing support for the health decisions of your community, empowering the people who are trying to make their family or neighborhood a healthier place to live. You are empowered when you and the doctor set an agenda together for the visit; in the same way, your community should set an agenda for promoting health.

You are empowered when you feel confident in communicating your preferences about your heath to your physician; your community should be able to communicate "within itself" and with health care professionals and public health workers.

You are empowered when you feel your emotions being taken into account, not just your decision making, in the context of medical decisions. In the same way, your community should be able to express itself, that is, to let the powers that be know about the worries, fears, and struggles that motivate it, so that the community can act with the best interest of its constituents at heart.

You are empowered when you are able to voice your priorities. Not everyone approaches their health care in the same way. Some people want aggressive treatment no matter what the adverse effects, as long as it seems to be in accord with the doctor's explicit or implicit preference; others would rather avoid anything that smacks of medical establishment or modern technologies whatever; and a large silent majority in the middle would just as soon do what the doctor says, if it seems reasonable, as long as it's not associated with significant inconvenience, cost, or danger—providing the condition is not life threatening (and if it is, then all bets are off).

We are empowered when we are recognized as individuals. Communities can be recognized as independent entities worthy of consideration, but that assumes that people identify themselves with a community. Not everyone does so. Not everyone who seems to be of a certain ethnicity (e.g., African American) actually identifies with that ethnicity. And those who might not seem to have much in common with a particular group might identify with it after all.

And even if a person identifies with a community, that community might have bigger problems than just health. It might be outside the members' power to do anything to help the most deep-rooted issues. The community I am thinking about is one I am familiar with as a doctor and resident of Baltimore, though only in a second-hand way: the African-American community. A number of my patients are from families that struggle with generational poverty. You might know or be part of such a family—even if you enjoy relative economic stability, you might have relatives whom you have to support, or who have health problems of their own. What is the best way to intervene? The answer is outside the bailiwick of health but essential to improving the health of so many, and the weakness of any approach that talks glibly about individuals, communities, and relationships.

WORKING WITH COMMUNITIES, UNDERSTANDING THEIR LIMITATIONS

It is not an easy matter to identify the problems that require an approach on the community level. This goes back to an ongoing division among different kinds of public health interventions. Do we—and our communities—respond to targeted measures that aim to change our behavior (e.g., ads about exercise, smoking cessation, and obesity)? Or is it government legislation and regulation that change our tune (e.g., cigarette taxes and limitations on the allowable sizes of sugary drinks)?

The two work together. Only when our community sees a problem as something to work on will it welcome the intervention of a government agency. Public health workers know this, which is why a community affected by a law needs to be educated about the reasons for that law—otherwise the intervention might be a failure even before it starts. Take a fundamentalist community like the ultra-Orthodox Jews, a subset of whom, or their leaders, believe that the Law of Moses requires that the circumciser, the mohel, place his mouth directly on the baby's penis to suck out blood. This ritual, called "metzitzah be-peh," is controversial.

The approach of the New York City Department of Health and Mental Hygiene (DOHMH) is instructive.[10] Clearly, having such mohels perform such a procedure is detrimental to the public's health, since it can transmit herpes along with other infectious diseases. Just as clearly, a public health agency in a democracy is loath to march in and demand that an isolated community change deep seated religious-ritual behavior for public health reasons, unless there is serious danger.

In this case, however, there was serious danger, and children did die. Why then did the New York City health officials not immediately outlaw such a religious procedure? There were some who called for such a move, including bioethicists,[11] but the DOHMH chose a different tack, that is, to talk to the leaders of the community and strike a balance between health and cooperation. I am of two minds about this approach, especially because the ultra-Orthodox community leadership is not democratically elected and includes rabbis and others whose view of science and medicine is obscurantist.

LEGISLATING HEALTH? EXAMPLES AND UNINTENDED CONSEQUENCES

Considering the importance in which certain rabbis held the ritual, the DOHMH thought it better to cooperate rather than heavy-handedly legislate. It is still unclear whether this approach was more effective than a more one-sided one would have been, but it does make us think about the downsides of public health legislation that affects other communities.

If, for example, my community includes many people who frequently consume 16-ounce sugared drinks, and the city forbids that such a size be sold, will people stop drinking those extra-large drinks, or will they merely get them from somewhere else? And, as a result, will a community's view of doctors, public health workers, and health strategies as a whole be affected?

There are public health issues for which we know that legislation does work. There are few ways to deliver tobacco, and if cigarettes are outlawed or taxed, it stands to reason that their consumption will decrease, to the benefit of the health of many communities. If you understand legislation as a tool to achieve public health goals, then pretty soon many problems in public health tend to look like nails for which legislation is a convenient hammer. In some cases the evidence lags the legislation. The effort to legislate the salt and saturated-fat content of restaurant menus is one such instance. Randomized controlled trials of low-salt diets have failed to show an impact on cardiovascular outcomes. Nor is it clear whether the efforts to reduce fat or sugar consumption will improve outcomes.[12]

Thus, there are conditions that require a more multifaceted strategy than that used for circumcisions, cigarette smoking, or vaccinations. Perhaps the number one disease that is most often labeled a public health epidemic is diabetes. Its prevalence is growing;[13] it leads to a wide variety of disabling conditions (not to mention death), and there is a growing consensus about how best to approach it. But this consensus might be missing an important element—that of the community.

COMMUNITY CARE AND DIABETES

A number of studies have already established the benefit of team treatment in diabetes: not just you and the doctor, but the nurse and the diabetes educator. These elements are not carved in stone: if not a nurse or a diabetes educator, then a health coach, someone who fills the role of a communicator that the doctor should be able to fill (as we have discussed above). Diabetes and blood sugar are controlled with more precision when the diabetes educator helps guide you. The educator and other members of the treatment team help not just in adherence to recommended diabetes treatment, but with coping mechanisms when life difficulties inevitably get in the way of checking blood sugar or self-administering insulin.[14]

But why do such treatment plans not explicitly include members of your community? We can imagine guides to managing diabetes that include not just you, the doctor, and the coach, but your family, friends, and community, each party with its defined role. For example, your parents or children might function as your reminders and pit crew as you face the day-to-day difficulties of life with a taxing disease, and strike that balance between coddling and pushing that parents and children have to manage.

In addition, we can change the culture of the community where diabetes is a problem, not just through public service announcements but through incentives at all levels: schools incorporating exercise, gardens providing food to local markets, and markets providing ways to get healthy food into the hands of those who need it, for example the elderly, the poor, parents and children.

Incentives can make it easier to put society on the path that promotes health, and I will talk in the next chapters about building a health-care system that respects our emotional needs in a relationship with our providers. Incentives won't work, however, without a society for them to act upon, or, other way around, for a society to act in response to them.

How can you and your community act for the sake of health in the context of diabetes?

1. Educate yourself, your friends, and family—whether or not you have the disease. An educated community can help its members.[15]
2. Find out whether your community offers convenient locations for physical exercise, even for a physical activity as simple as walking. Walking can improve control of blood sugar[16] but for many people it is difficult to find a space to walk in. Even if you can't create a park where none exists, you can walk at your workplace, a mall, or in a school.
3. Discuss the availability of healthy food with popular restaurants in your area.

4. Research the quality, availability, and patient-centeredness of doctors and hospitals to the members of your community. If, for example, the people you know speak a language that is not understood or interpreted by local health care providers, it doesn't seem likely that they will be able to have a concrete and direct discussion with you about diabetes.

If your hospitals or doctors are not addressing the needs of your community, you need to let them know. Many of us are not comfortable in the role of strident agitator or even quiet advocate. However, if there is some information that certain practitioners or hospitals are more open to your community than others, you should choose them.

DOES COMMUNITY EMPOWERMENT ACTUALLY WORK?

Wait, you might say. What does it matter what doctor or hospital you go to, when the main thing is getting the right medical attention when you need it? It doesn't matter whom you see, as long as they do the right job. As we have discussed above, the evidence for choosing doctors or hospitals presented now to the public is incomplete in important respects, but in any case one can make this objection to many of the claims made in this book: effectiveness is the key, and focusing on personality or relationships is misguided.

I acknowledge that for some of the interventions I have discussed, and certainly those on the broad scale of communities, the effectiveness is untested. I cannot confidently say that basing your relationship with the doctor on a stable footing of good communication, and extending that communicativeness to the community, will drop everyone's blood pressure to healthy levels and cure everyone's diabetes.

That assumes, however, that encouraging health care that is responsive to communities can be effective in only one way: through immediately improving control or treatment of a given disease.

Empowering our communities can have a number of other positive effects: through strengthening the connection between our neighborhoods and our doctors; making sure our objections, problems, and queries are met; and, most fundamentally, making sure that we are on the same page as our health care providers regarding the outcomes that matter to us.

There are important health outcomes that matter to everyone: death, disability, and hospitalization. But people differ on what "price" they would pay to achieve them (e.g., what quality of life they would give up, what inconvenient, expensive, or deleterious medications they would subject themselves to). For example, some men with prostate cancer would choose a therapeutic regimen that guarantees less than maximum survival if their sexual potency would not be reduced.[17] Years off a life for an erection: only with a frank discussion and open communication between doctor and patient can that trade-off be made with open eyes.

People also differ regarding how aggressive they would like their doctors to be and how much disruption they are willing to tolerate in their lives. There is a growing realization that more aggressive medical treatment, more tests, more procedures, and more medicine are not necessarily better for us, and better communication can make this realization clearer to both parties in the medical encounter. The next chapter will talk about this.

Chapter Thirteen

Learning How to Want Less: Creating a Resource-Sparing Medical Culture Together with Our Doctors

DIFFERENCES OF OPINION: IS MORE CARE BETTER?

I went to a lecture recently at Johns Hopkins by two esteemed physicians from Harvard Medical School, Jerome Groopman and Pamela Hartzband, who were discussing the cognitive biases of doctors and physicians. [1]

As part of their lecture, they talked about an area of wide disagreement: whether men should undergo regular screening for prostate cancer. As I mentioned earlier in this book, one study in Europe showed that mortality was decreased in a small way by such screening; however, a similar study in the United States did not reach such a conclusion. A more recent trial showed that prostatectomy as a reaction to prostate-cancer screening did not improve death rates from prostate cancer over twelve years of follow-up. [2]

On the basis of a small number of such studies, the recommendations of several leading professional organizations contradict each other about the utility of prostate cancer screening. The United States Preventive Services Task Force (USPSTF) recommends against routine prostate cancer screening using the prostate specific antigen (PSA) blood test. [3] On the other hand, the American Cancer Society recommends that doctor and patient discuss it, and explicitly recommends early screening for prostate cancer in certain circumstances. [4]

Drs. Groopman and Hartzband came to the conclusion that the cognitive or other biases of these various organizations partially drove their decision making. The urologists and oncologists come from a culture of aggressive treatment, while the internists and clinical epidemiologists (represented, by and large, by the USPSTF) suggest that not everyone needs aggressive screening.

But treating, screening, and prescribing less aggressively is not merely another cognitive bias. Our health care system is focused on aggressive use of technologies, rapid uptake of unproven new devices and widespread prescription of medications that might or might not help.[5]

Examples of this tendency, which is so deeply ingrained in our American medical system as to be a characteristic and not merely a worrying trend, are legion. Common conditions, such as lower back pain, are rife with the overuse of advanced imaging, like CT scans and MRIs, which helps precious few people, costs millions of dollars a year, and can lead to unnecessary surgery even when surgery is not indicated.[6]

This last point is not meant to blame the surgeons. When an MRI is used, chances are that the radiologist will not find anything "normal": the imaging technology is sensitive enough to pick up characteristics that might never be seen on a "less sensitive" X-ray or CT scan; unfortunately, many of these characteristics are not relevant at all to our back pain. We can have an MRI, which shows something in our back that never existed before, and then see a surgeon for the repair of that "defect" which might have nothing to do with our pain and thus, bring no benefit when repaired.

This example repeats itself time and time again for many different health problems, as if in a funhouse mirror. High blood pressure has been defined down for decades; that is, the value of blood pressure at which hypertension is diagnosed has slid to ever lower values. For people with diabetes, we are told, the blood pressure should be 130/80. For people with kidney disease, perhaps a little bit lower. But there is little evidence that blood pressures under 140/90 come with better health outcomes. Nonetheless, more blood pressure medications are being marketed and prescribed.[7]

OVERUSE IN BACK PAIN: ARE WE THE PROBLEM?

To return to the first example of back pain, why do many patients do not see that the fixes so often proffered—joint injections, surgery, electronic devices—are often not worth the expense, invasiveness, or recuperation after the procedure?

Because we patients are part of the problem. Sure, there are doctors who recommend courses of treatment that might not help, some of them doing so because they have a financial interest. There are specialists who stand to gain from imaging technologies, and big pharmaceutical firms that make money off analgesics and other medications to treat back pain.

But we are the ones who end up going along with these ill-advised treatments, more often than not. Our intentions are understandable and even laudable—we want our pain to be treated, we assume. But do we? Is that the only thing we want when we realize we have back pain?

Sure we want it to go away, but not at any price. There have been studies done on the people's approaches to their back pain, and their motivations are not limited to making the pain go away. They want their pain to be appreciated, and their own stories to be heard in the context of a respectful, equitable relationship with the doctor.[8] Even if their doctor is technically proficient at performing a procedure meant to reduce their back pain, something is missing if he or she does not demonstrate empathy.

The flip side is also true: if we have a doctor who can tell us that back pain is common, it usually goes away by itself in any case, and the procedures and medicine do not furnish a risk free or certain cure even when the pain might become chronic, we might be able to accept that bad news by virtue of the relationship that I have been talking about throughout this book. We might be better able to accept the ups and downs of a chronic condition when there is someone to weather them with us. And if that person, our doctor, is prepared with the information to balance risk and benefits so that we can be supported in our decision making, so much the better.

Back pain might be an easier example to make this case, bringing to bear the power of the relationship on a condition that accounts for a considerable amount of overtreatment and overuse. While advanced imaging technologies (CT scans and MRIs) account for millions of dollars of costs, and back pain is a common condition, it is not the most terrible of the diseases we fear. What do we do when we are faced with conditions for which there is no proven treatment? Can we look death in the face and fight it with weapons that are proven effective, not therapy that might be as bad as any disease?

A recent study in the *New England Journal of Medicine* lays out the facts of our perception of cancer treatment in those with advanced disease. Sixty-nine percent of patients with metastatic lung cancer and 81 percent of those with metastatic colorectal cancer did not understand that chemotherapy was not going to cure their cancer.[9] Many times we ask for treatments on the basis of a misperception of their effectiveness. We have a mistaken faith in the powers of medicine and think that all disease might be treatable—or curable.

WHAT IF OUR HEALTH PROBLEMS AREN'T TREATABLE?

How much of what we suffer from is curable? Much more than used to be the case. Infectious diseases have been wiped out or made susceptible to treatment, though death rates due to these diseases have actually increased in recent years.[10] Mortality due to heart attacks has decreased about four-fold over the past sixty years. We can even prevent heart attacks by controlling cardiac risk factors.[11] HIV, thirty years ago a death sentence, is now a chronic illness for those lucky enough to have access to medications and treatments, though it is associated with decreased life expectancy and an increased risk of certain other diseases, for example, heart disease.[12] Certain forms of cancer are now widely screened, for example cervical cancer, and as a result the mortality associated with them has decreased.

For many other problems, however, our arsenal is still incomplete. In the case of diabetes, we know that most people in the outpatient setting use methods of insulin delivery that are inefficient and unpleasant. While insulin pumps, and "artificial pancreases" which combine real-time blood sugar sensing and continuous insulin delivery, are available, they are expensive, kludgey (made up of poorly matched components), and not usually covered by insurance.

Still other problems are not yet fully understood, and therapies are a generation, if that, away from becoming widely effective and available. In this case, I am talking about depression, a common ailment for which, you might think, dozens of medications are available. However, the best study available on the natural history of treated depression shows that such medications are effective about half the time,[13] and some literature indicates that therapy is oftentimes as effective as the medications.[14] This literature is limited because there is no economic incentive to conduct long, complicated trials that compare treatment with medication against treatment with therapy.

IF WE MAKE THE DECISION, WILL WE WANT LESS?

If treatment doesn't do as much as we think, and if we are misinformed about the extent to which our health problem is susceptible to treatment, maybe we'll want less. And perhaps if we as patients are put in control of the decision making, we will naturally decide to have less to do with complicated, invasive, and expensive treatments and tests.

Equipping us as patients for shared decision making is currently gaining in popularity. This is a salutary trend, because if we are enabled to discuss options as near equals with the doctor, rather than as subordinates, our relationship might be on a better footing and we might be able to make decisions that more reflect our preferences.

However, as more and more decisions are made according to the principles of shared decision making, an increasing number of them will run up against situations where there is not enough information an informed decision, or no effective treatment is available. We will lack reliable guidance.

What should we do in those cases? Obviously, we have to be satisfied with the limited information available, and we have to make a choice. But even in making such a choice with incomplete information, we should be cognizant of what it means to choose aggressive therapies.

WHAT AGGRESSIVE THERAPIES CAN DO

Cost. Certainly, if we are lucky enough to be insured, we will often not pay the full cost of the procedures and treatments recommended to us. Insured patients are often not even aware of the real cost, since this information is not available. While there are initiatives afoot to show doctors and patients the true cost of the interventions contemplated when a medical decision is made, they are few and still getting off the ground. The cost is passed on to our employers, hospitals, insurers, and the federal government. Our country spends more on health care and gets less than other countries,[15] and more money on health care means less spent on other societal needs.

Picking physical therapy rather than imaging for back pain will save hundreds of millions of dollars a year, but since the total health care expenditures yearly in the United States amount to more than two trillion dollars yearly, this will not save our budgetary bacon. There is, however, the tantalizing possibility that incremental change to favor doing less and choosing wisely might, over time, move the needle to a health care system which respects cost constraints and orders only the tests and treatments that work.

There are huge solutions envisioned as part of governmental health care reform, which were designed to change payment mechanisms, thus encouraging doctors toward certain interventions and not others. But such top-down interventions, such as the Independent Payment Advisory Board envisioned as part of the Affordable Care Act, might backfire because many people just don't understand why more costly treatments aren't necessarily better; thus we might ask for them anyway. Which brings us to the next point to make about aggressive therapies.

Effectiveness. It does not make sense to pursue more aggressive treatments or testing modalities until you can be sure they will find something worth the extra aggravation. Often, however, the scan or the test is done because the doctor has a technology to do it (so-called supply-driven demand).[16] The MRI does not make back pain better, surgery does not improve many kinds of chronic pain, and the CT scan doesn't do much good if you are eating two meals a day consisting entirely of soda and fried foods. Doing a scan to "find out what is going on" makes just as much sense as a mechanic changing your oil as an automatic response to any car problem. We want something done that works, not merely because the technology is the latest and greatest thing.

Effectiveness means defining what matters to you as a person and to people like you and figuring out what the scientific literature says, or doesn't say, and how those results match up to the outcomes that matter by making sure that your situation and the treatments or tests planned can be compared to any promising findings in the literature. Often only a minority of these criteria are met. Statistical measures meant to represent our quality of life are not the same thing as our own perceived quality of life, and our preferences need not match with them. [17] If we are the sort of person who, for any one of a number of possible reasons, would not be eligible for a research study—either because of our other health problems, or just because of our race, ethnicity, age, or sex—perhaps those research findings do not apply to us.

Thus, if a doctor is trying to recommend a treatment to us, we should not decide whether it might work for us without asking specific questions and being careful in our expectations. We should always ask, "How might the research studies apply to me as a person? Are we sure that the benefits or side effects will be in a favorable balance for me?" An honest physician should be able to say, "I am not sure"—but give some reasoned speculation.

ADVERSE EFFECTS

I try not to call these effects "side effects" because they don't happen off on the side, in some unimportant corner, but right at the center of the life of the affected person. Doctors' language even de-emphasizes the importance of adverse effects; doctors say for example "the patient discontinued the medication; she could not tolerate it due to side effects." Toleration, as if lack of character made a person unable to put up with the fatigue of beta blockers prescribed for coronary artery disease, or with the low blood sugar caused by some diabetes medications.

Adverse effects are wider and deeper than people often admit. A medication can make us feel worse and can lead to considerable cost and inconvenience, of course, but it can also interact with the other medications that one is already taking, leading in turn to more symptoms that the doctor often does not correctly attribute to medications. Furthermore, once a medication is started, whether or not its effectiveness was well founded for the condition it was given for, we presume that the condition is in fact one that should be treated with medications.

ADVERSE EFFECTS, MEDICATIONS, AND THE VICIOUS CYCLE: A STORY

A concrete example might make these ideas clearer. I have a patient from Finland, Mr. Rose, in his forties (I have changed identifying details). He came to his cardiologist reporting palpitations. It is important to know that

Mr. Rose has a lot of problems, chronic pain, and many surgeries to show for it.

Had he come to see me before he saw his cardiologists, I would have recommended that we follow his arrhythmia rather than embark on any new course of testing or treatment. In this case, unfortunately, if I had seen him first, I would have been right that an intervention for this problem might lead to more harm than good.

He was taken to the electrophysiology laboratory, where cardiologists try to analyze the characteristics of abnormal heart rhythms. Such procedures are generally indicated for abnormal rhythms that can lead to serious health consequences, such as atrial fibrillation, which can be associated with blood clots, or ventricular tachycardia, which can cause death. His rhythm was not found to be one of these problematic rhythms. So far so good: electrophysiologists and their equipment can do wonders for preventing such nefarious rhythms and the problems they cause.

He reported pain and was terribly anxious after the procedure—one adverse effect of the intervention. Afterwards, however, the gentleman still wanted some medication to treat his rhythm. So they gave him one.

Several months later, he came to my office reporting fatigue and leg swelling. I took a look; indeed, his legs were swollen to far more than their normal size. I could sink my finger into them and watch the dimples remain for a good few seconds. Seeing such swollen legs makes anyone's heart skip a beat, and I knew that something had to be wrong. No one had to tell him that, either.

There are times when the physical exam is more suspenseful than it should be. The patient had shown me his legs, but now I had to go over the rest of his body. His neck veins were not swollen and there did not appear to be any abnormalities on his heart exam. Later, an X-ray showed no extra fluid and an echocardiography (ultrasound) of his heart showed that it was pumping normally, with no decreased motion. All this together made me confident that his heart was not the problem. Nor, as future lab tests showed, were his thyroid or iron level (problems which can cause fatigue) the issue. He did not have any blood clots in his lungs or his legs.

Regretfully, I had to conclude that, with all other possible factors having been eliminated, the most likely guilty party here was the medication he had been given for his heart rhythm.

In hindsight, it wasn't certain to me that he should have gotten such a medication at all. Perhaps treating his chronic pain would have slowed down his heart rhythm just the same. This would not have been a quick fix, since he has had such pain for years, but at least it would not have saddled him with tests, treatments, and side effects to get through.

I picked up the phone, but when I told him what I thought was going on, the response was not what I was expecting. "Well, I am talking to the cardiologists tomorrow and they will tell me what tests I need to do," he said. "I am not sure you need any more tests," I said. "I think the medication is the culprit." "But I know something is wrong," he persisted.

Clearly I was not getting through to him. Where did I go wrong? I thought about it after our phone conversation had come to a mercifully quick end. It wasn't that I knew more than him, and I was failing to get across my superior knowledge and medical acumen. Rather, this instance symbolized the failure of a health-care system. He felt like something was wrong that I was not addressing.

I tried using what junior doctors used to call, during a residency program in primary care, "psychosocial judo": all the communication techniques that I have been preaching for the length of this book. I told him, "I can see that you are really bothered by this." I flatter myself that I am a pretty good listener, and I took care to use open body language to show that I was engaged in the conversation. When I had seen the patient in person, when those swollen legs were the topic of conversation, I even asked him what he thought we should do. He said, frustratingly, "You're the doctor."

Now, after the tests I had recommended, here we were, up against a solution that he did not find satisfactory. I had tried telegraphing my care and attention to his problem, but he did not agree that the medicine was causing his symptoms.

As I write this, I am still in the middle of the story. I don't know what further treatments or tests Mr. Rose will pursue in order to find out, as he has been saying, "what is really going on." But I do know that his desire to get to the bottom of the thing is related less to a desire for causal clarity than for an instinct to "do everything."

This instinct is itself a weighty adverse effect, driving much of the unfounded expenditure, procedures, testing, and treatments of our health system. For Mr. Rose, it is too late to reassure him. In fact, as I have been writing these words, he has decided to leave me and see another doctor who might be ready to order more tests and procedures. I did not convince him that I was listening to his symptoms.

He has already made his choice, and been formed in a system where "do another test" is the answer to a health problem whose cause is not immediately clear. Perhaps, however, in a future generation, or in pockets of our health care system where overuse is being addressed, we can change that conception of what medicine is supposed to do for us.

CHANGING THE CULTURE: VARIATION IN CARE AND OVERUSE

This category perhaps overlaps somewhat with the previous two, but it underlies both of them. Mr. Rose has learned to expect additional tests, treatments, and procedures as a sign that the doctor cares about his problem. The doctor has learned that ordering another test is always accepted as a sign that she is still looking into things, that patients have not been abandoned.

By the same token, the doctors have been socialized, acculturated, and incentivized to go farther and farther afield. Part of the reason has been dissected by researchers at Dartmouth College [18] who have compared the amount of health care expenditure in the last months of life among different medical centers. They compare those months of life so as to control for differences in people or their diseases which might bias the results. They found that the health care costs vary remarkably from region to region, and even from hospital to hospital.

What can possibly explain this variation? Why is a hospital like NYU's Tisch near the top of the list, and other hospitals in the same city at the bottom? The full answers are still being pieced together, and there are researchers who claim that the difference in health-care costs can still be explained by differences in patients or their disease severity. [19] But the Dartmouth researchers show that at least part of the difference is supply sided: that is, the more technologies, tests, and treatments are available, the more often they tend to be used.

Some of this variation has to do with economic incentives. Many doctors' practices own medical equipment, such as scanners, and many doctor's associations are now in partnership with hospitals where many specialists and their equipment are located, which provides an obvious incentive to order such tests. But even beyond such cold economics, our entire system of medical education provides incentives to test and treat without particular attention to their effectiveness. Specialists exist not just because of their special fund of knowledge but because they are the gatekeepers for special tests. Our system emphasizes the training and compensation of specialists over that of primary care doctors and family practice doctors, as well as other practitioners who consider the care of the whole patient, like nurse practitioners and physician assistants.

It becomes a vicious cycle, or a snake of overuse eating its tail. As tests, imaging, and treatments become available, they are used, whether or not they are proven effective. One example of this is the phenomenon of off-label use. [20] Medications approved by the Food and Drug Administration for one use are used for another condition without due consideration, and often even without discussion with the person who might be using the medication, as to whether they might work for the new indication.

"A BATTERY OF TESTS": WHEN SCREENING TESTS DON'T WORK

Another example of such overuse is the attitude many patients take toward screening tests. Such tests are ideally supposed to find early signs of a condition that is reasonably frequent in the population, detectable by the test itself, and susceptible to cure or treatment if found. However, as more and more tests become available, the connection of some of them to diseases that matter to us becomes more and more tenuous.

Let's take the example of blood tests for cholesterol, which have been broadly available as an automated test for about thirty-five years.[21] In that time, they have become one of the most commonly ordered blood tests. The next time your doctor suggests that you have a lipid panel, you might ask him or her why. The answer is likely to be something like, "Cholesterol levels increase the risk of heart disease." This is true. Few doctors would disagree with the importance of elevated cholesterol as a contributor to the chance that you might develop a heart attack.

However, the devil of overuse is in the details. How often should a cholesterol panel be repeated? What are the values of "good cholesterol" (HDL) and "bad cholesterol" (LDL) for which treatment with medications, rather than diet and exercise, are recommended? Do cholesterol medications protect someone from heart disease better than diet and exercise, if both get you to the same cholesterol numbers?

There are multiple similar questions for each one of the dozens of tests that might typically be ordered during a doctor's visit. But for most tests, patients don't know the most basic information: how often tests should be done; what the numbers mean; or whether therapy with medications or procedures significantly improves results over conservative therapy or watchful waiting.

I have been part of an initiative to try and reverse this trend. The initiative was the "Top 5" project of the National Physicians Alliance, an advocacy group for patient-centered care among primary care physicians. Under the leadership of Stephen Smith, we convened focus groups among physicians to ask them about the procedures or tests that were most often done without clear benefit for the patient.

We came up with a number of candidates but eventually settled on a list of five tests: electrocardiograms done in people without heart symptoms; MRIs for back pain; urine tests or tests of electrolytes (metabolic panels) in people without symptoms, and bone mineral scans in women under 65 years old or without risk factors for bone disease. If your doctor has recommended one of these tests to you as a screening test, you should ask him for more information about why he thinks it's indicated.[22]

Doctors in the specialties of internal medicine, family practice, and pediatrics assembled lists; the second stage of the initiative has currently begun: small monetary incentives are being provided to practices that can show lower rates of use of these overused tests among their residents (junior doctors). The American College of Physicians, an important professional group, assembled a larger list on the same principles. [23]

REDUCING OVERUSE THROUGH THE RELATIONSHIP

What these initiatives lack, however, is a mechanism to reduce contraindicated testing on the basis of the relationship between us and our doctors. Based upon the principles I have already discussed, a good conversation between us and our doctors does not begin with the name of a test that a doctor is planning on ordering. It begins with a discussion between us and our doctors about our concerns and a negotiation of the agenda. Sure, the doctor might have a different list of things she considers important than we do, but we should be able to come around to an agreement on a common set of problems that we can address. Such a negotiation of agenda, which is dependent on a working relationship and effective communication, can help ameliorate the problem of overuse in three ways:

1. If we can talk to the doctor about our concerns, we might not ask for a test in order to achieve the reassurance that is missing.
2. If the doctor can talk to us about the history of our problem, the doctor might not order a test to "find out what is going on" because he might have found it out already by talking to us and doing a physical exam.
3. If we maintain a relationship with our regular doctor, we do not have to have recourse to an ever-changing lineup of specialists each time we feel symptoms in another region of our body.

Let me be clear about the esteem in which I hold specialists. Many patients would not have their symptoms addressed, or their health improved, without them. The neurologists who treat seizures and nerve pain, or Parkinson's Disease; the cardiologist who unblocks our blood vessels or fixes our heart rhythm; the gastroenterologist who quiets the inflammation of our Crohn's disease; the psychiatrist who fine-tunes our therapy and pharmacological regimen—all these people are essential to health.

They are essential only in the right context, however. There is little guidance available for doctors or patients about when to have recourse to specialists and when to take care of the concern in the context of the already existing doctor-patient relationship. As with much else, doctors and patients use referral to a specialist as a way to show that the concern of the patient is being addressed, without necessarily any particular request or question for the specialist.

If ordering tests or images or referrals to specialists is often done out of an unclear sense of "doing something to help" (without a well-thought-out list of questions that these tests are meant to answer and without any strong basis in the scientific evidence), why do we still want to order them? We can blame the perverted economic incentives of our health care system and doctors' tendencies to order tests first and check the evidence later, or pharmaceutical and medical technology firms' vested interest in popularizing such tests.

The fact is though that patients want them, too. We don't feel right if we go to a doctor without blood tests, a prescription, or a referral for an appointment. My hope is that the cultural change represented by programs to reduce overuse will percolate down to us and our doctors. If we hear our doctors telling us the bad things that can happen from a test that isn't indicated, and we share our own reservations with our doctors, perhaps we can ground more of our care in the mutual understanding of a relationship rather than the quick fix of an additional test.

This prediction of a change in culture is aspirational. Whether a cultural change toward relationship and communication and away from reflexive testing and referring is at all realistic is connected to a broader conversation that has been held recently in the lay press: how is health care change to be carried out? Should it be wholesale, as advocates of single-payer systems might want, or incremental?

In either case, change on the level of doctor and patient is not enough. We need some form of health system change. The Patient Protection and Affordable Care Act (Obamacare), while a great start, is not the complete package. We need to found an improved health system on improved communication and relationships over time. In the next and final chapter, I will outline a plan for doing that.

Chapter Fourteen

Transforming Our Health Care System Through Communication and Collaboration

I have learned a lot about health care through social media, including Twitter, and met people I never would have talked to in my circumscribed real world. One group I have become well acquainted with is the hundreds if not thousands of patient advocates. Their slogan, in a nutshell, is "Give me my damn data!"[1] According to the previous paternalistic model of medicine, patients are more acted on than they are actors. But according to the patient-centered model, patients drive the process of care. "Nothing about me, without me,"[2] is the phrase, and it makes sense. Patient-centered care makes each one of us the center of the medical encounter with our doctor, and thus responsible for the collection of data and, perhaps, even medical decision making.

But do we want that decision making? Not everyone does.[3] Indeed, we go to doctors because we want to discuss decisions with them. Many of us assume perhaps that the doctor will make the decision in any case; what matters is how the doctor behaves with us while he is she is doing so.[4] If not everyone is comfortable making their own medical decisions, do the many patient advocates place an unwanted burden on those who do not want the responsibilities?

We should also consider who these patient advocates are. They are net natives, denizens of social media. They are fluent in accessing and manipulating data, and they take for granted a comfort with that data that not everyone has.

WHEN IT'S DIFFICULT TO ADVOCATE FOR YOURSELF

It's easy to preach about emotional and intellectual readiness, agenda setting, and mind-meeting to those who have the world on a string and a tablet computer on their lap. But there are those—no less intelligent—who lack resources, whether here in the United States or elsewhere. Who is the advocate for these patients, and what if, in the end, they do not want to make medical decisions or even be at the center of the doctor-patient encounter?

We need to consider three barriers many of us face in making our medical decisions. Even if the barriers are removed, we might not want to make the decisions. And it is not obvious, in the end, that the ideal health care system is structured around our own medical decision making. I will consider the three barriers in turn.

First, think about the difficulties you might be facing in your own life. You might, for example, have come to the United States from another country not too many months ago, and do not speak English. Any clinic receiving Medicare or Medicaid is required by law to provide interpreter services to anyone of low English proficiency,[5] but you don't know that. All you know is that when you are called in to see the doctor, she asks your daughter, who is with you, to translate, and all of a sudden you find you are a lot less enthusiastic to talk about the problem you came with.

Or imagine yourself in another possible situation: you have been unemployed for a long time, and you have terrible back pain that won't go away. You would love for there to be something you could do about it. The doctor tells you that physical therapy is the best available option; getting an MRI won't change much, unless you decide to do surgery, which might not help. But the physical therapy clinic is located some distance from where you live, is not completely covered by insurance, and requires a referral from a primary care physician, which you don't have.

Third, you are one of the many Americans who are taking care of other people's children because their parents are sick, in jail, or abusing alcohol or drugs.

If you are one of these types of people, how are you supposed to be an effective self-advocate or own "your data" enough to be capable of making your medical decisions? Apart from these kinds of barriers, there is another group of difficulties that tends to go along with them, but not always. You might be someone who is lucky enough to be employed; your family is healthy, and you have enough money and family support. All of a sudden, however, you find out that you might need an operation and you don't know the first thing about it. The doctor puts a list of options in front of you: you have a spot on the liver, and there are multiple possible procedures. She can cut it out, or inject something into it, or do a couple of other things. You don't understand the terms she uses. The doctor tells you what the risks of each procedure are, but you have no idea how much trust to put in her words. The risks scare and confuse you, though you have never thought of yourself as an unintelligent person.

Or, to take a final example, you are a woman who went through menopause a few years ago. You are now 58 years old and you have been told by your doctor that a special kind of X-ray, a bone mineral scan, "was necessary" to estimate the risk of developing a bone fracture in "a few years." You weren't sure, to be honest, how convinced you were about the necessity of the scan, but you liked the doctor so went ahead with it anyway. Now you have been called into her office to talk about the results. "So we did the DEXA scan," she says to you. "The what?" you respond. "The bone mineral scan. And I wanted to talk to you about the results." You shake your head okay, and she proceeds to show you a sheet with lines full of numbers, though you were never good at math in school. She says something about T scores and Z scores but quickly seems to realize that your eyes are glazing over.

"So I feed these numbers into a model which we often use, and I come up with the ten-year probability that you might have a hip fracture, together with the ten-year probability you might have any fracture from osteoporosis." You recognize that word, and ask if you do, in fact, have osteoporosis. Yes, she confirms. Then she goes on about the ten-year probabilities. She says you have a 4 percent probability over the next ten years of having a hip fracture, and a 15 percent probability over the next ten years of having any fracture due to osteoporosis.

You ask her, what it means to have a fracture sometime in the next ten years, and how someone figures out the chance of that. You really are concentrating on today, not years from now. You have children and grandchildren to take care of; you are working two jobs, one in the morning for the city department of social services, the other in the evening for a cleaning company. If you had a bone fracture now, that would upend your world. On the other hand, you don't know how to figure out whether you are going to have a fracture ten years from now. What does that even mean? You ask the doctor how to understand those numbers, but you are worried that she thinks you are an idiot. And since this is the first time you are meeting her, you don't want her to think you a bad patient who won't follow instructions.

HEALTH CARE COSTS AND THE CARE OF THE SICKEST

I have no ironclad proof for the argument of this chapter, but each of the following statements is backed up by rock-solid facts.

The poorest and most disadvantaged of our society are the sickest. Obviously, this is a burden to them as individuals. But the effect of their ill health ripples outward to their friends, families, and whole communities.[6] These sickest patients require treatment, and this treatment costs money. However, their care does not represent the most important cause of the increase in health care costs in the United States. On the contrary, health care costs are increasing for reasons that have little to do with treating our sickest, most disadvantaged citizens.

Up to 20 percent of health care costs, as detailed in a recent article in the *Journal of the American Medical Association*, comes from imperfections of our system which do not benefit the patient at all.[7] But through building a productive relationship with the physician, we can help address those imperfections, and play a role as individuals in decreasing the burden on the American budget of health care costs.

How would this work? The 20 percent comes from waste and overuse, which Donald Berwick and Andrew Hackbarth divide into six categories: "overtreatment, failures of care coordination, failures in execution of care processes, administrative complexity, pricing failures, and fraud and abuse." By focusing on the relationship with the primary care provider, we can favorably influence some of these categories and thus reduce this large chunk, more than one-fifth, of health care costs.

As for overtreatment, doctors and patients have recourse to expensive tests often because they are not sure what else to do,[8] or because they do not have time to explore the reasons for a complaint through the history or the physical exam.[9] Helping ferret out the causes of a problem takes time, and often multiple visits. When, for example, an MRI is used for garden-variety lower back pain without signs of a serious problem, the MRI will pick up "abnormalities" which are not clinically significant at all and do not have clear bearing on the pain. But the MRI shows an abnormality, and someone thinks we should follow up on it—and thus it starts, the vicious cycle of tests that lead to more tests without any point at which someone says stop.

There are other kinds of overtreatment. Very recently the *New England Journal of Medicine* published the results of a study that confirmed what many doctors had suspected for decades: mammograms do not actually save a significant number of lives. The drive for mammograms in all women over age fifty has become increasingly insistent, and a staple of breast-cancer advocacy organizations. The 2009 recommendations of the United States Preventive Services Task Force aroused controversy for their conclusion that mammograms for women between ages forty and fifty were not routinely justified, since about twice as many women in that age group needed to be screened to find one case of cancer as compared to women between 50 and 60 years of age.[10]

Lost in that discussion, however, was a more fundamental question: does universal breast cancer screening with mammograms save lives? The assumption all along was that imaging the breasts would show small abnormalities, undetectable by the woman or her doctor, which would be caught and treated before they were left to grow more dangerous—but also, in the bargain, that fewer late stage cancers would be found, since they would have been caught upstream by the screening test and removed before developing further.

The screening program only works if both ends are true. If more early-stage cancers are found without fewer late stage cancers being picked up, the screening test is detecting abnormalities that might not have affected health or lifespan. The *New England Journal* study found that the number of late-stage cancers found by screening mammography was decreased by only 8 per 100,000, perhaps not enough to make the entire machinery of screening worthwhile.[11]

IF SCREENING TESTS ARE IMPERFECT, WHAT IS OUR DOCTOR FOR?

Communication as the foundation of a relationship with your primary care provider could convert this overuse into appropriate use. As we have described in previous chapters, you should ideally be able to freely discuss with your doctor your feelings and fears about breast cancer, and how important it is to you. In return, your provider would be able to use those concerns of yours, together with information about your family history, to discuss your risk for developing breast cancer.

There are multiple models freely available for calculating that risk. So what is the point of cultivating such a relationship between us and our doctor when we can find the information ourselves on the Internet?[12] Because even at this late date, and with all the promised interconnectedness and open-data slogans of the Internet age, most people still have difficulties with applying the numbers of studies and models to their own lives.

Part of this is because we have difficulty with specialized concepts in health care or the world of numbers: health literacy and numeracy are the terms for these abilities. But the more fundamental reason for our difficulties is that the evidence never points to a single sure solution appropriate for you as an individual. Even if you have a high risk of breast cancer in your family, no flag is going to be thrown, no one is going to pin your arms behind your back and make you undergo a mammogram. It falls to you and your doctor to discuss the risks and benefits of breast imaging.

I used to think that it was our personal preferences that determine our health choices; today's impassioned patient advocates would agree with this. But if you don't have any relevant way to interpret the risk of breast cancer, how can you make the decision? Thus I would say now that the relationship between you and your provider bridges the gap between evidence and decision making. All evidence is incomplete and a decision is difficult to reach without help.

If you identify the decision that seems right to you, you are achieving treatment rather than overtreatment. You can never know if you are making exactly the right decision, but you can put it into the context of your interests and preferences, which your doctor is familiar with, and the ongoing history of your health care as part of the relationship.

A solid doctor-patient relationship can also help *failures of care coordination*. Care coordination is jargon for "health care professionals talking to each other." We have all experienced the ways in which doctors communicate, or fail to communicate, with each other. A doctor sends you to a specialist without telling either you or the specialist why he thinks this might be a good thing to do. This is particularly detrimental when both you and your doctor are trying to figure out a problem that has been bothering you for a long time, because the specialist can order a series of tests without considering the problem in context.

But care coordination means more than just telling the specialist why the primary care doctor is requesting the specialists' involvement. It means putting limits on the involvement beforehand, so that patients are not sucked in the maelstrom of test after test. It means, like in any successful relationship, delineating roles beforehand so that there are no misunderstandings.

Plenty of such misunderstandings arise in the course of patients being seen by a number of doctors. When a blood test is ordered by the specialist, but the results are available in the computer for a number of doctors, whose responsibility is it to communicate those results to us and explain what the results mean? The specialist assumes that, since we have already seen them in their office, completing as it were their tour of duty, the task falls to our primary care doctor; but the primary care doctor, often overwhelmed, reasonably assumed that the specialty physician who ordered the test will be the one to explain it to us. While currently it is up to us to clarify the roles of specialists and our primary care doctors (which one explains lab tests and the like) it shouldn't be that way. We should bring up this issue with our doctors so they can work it out. Communication might also aid in addressing so-called *failures in execution of care processes*. This means many things: for example, in the hospital, when the doctors recommend one medication but another is administered, or when, shockingly and not infrequently, the wrong limb is operated on. The many varieties, causes, and consequences of failures in hospital safety and quality have been well documented recently by my Johns Hopkins colleagues, Peter Pronovost and Eric Vohr[13] and Marty Makary.[14] In the outpatient setting too, however, the devil is in the details—or, to phrase it less felicitously, the execution of care processes can lead to problems.

Let's take, again, diabetes—so common, so supposedly "easy to treat" when doctors describe it, but a disease that can cause a myriad of problems because of, not despite, treatment. In about half of all patients with diabetes, recommended therapy is some sort of pill to reduce blood sugar or increase the body's sensitivity to diabetes; in the other half, insulin, the molecule that brings blood sugar into the cells, is recommended. But what might seem like a simple task can become confused in the application.

If we talk about pills, one medication, metformin, is nearly universally recommended as the best starting oral treatment for diabetes in patients who are otherwise healthy.[15] While there are a number of new diabetes medications, the evidence does not show that they are better than those already existing; in fact, in some instances they are worse.[16] Much of the diversity might have to do with the influence of pharmaceutical companies, which promote their favorite brand of medication. It is sobering to realize that the literature does not often answer a basic question: When diabetes can be treated with a pill, how often do doctors prescribe the most effective oral medication? If we have diabetes or know someone who does, it behooves us to be open with our doctor, asking her whether the medications given are the best ones for us.

With insulin, too, errors can be made, sometimes dangerous ones, and often due to a lack of communication with the primary care physician. Too much insulin can lead to dangerously low levels of blood sugar; too little, and the diabetes is barely scratched.

It stands to reason, then, that insulin treatment of diabetes is by no means a one-size-fits-all proposition. Sensitivity to insulin varies among people; increasing the dose the same amount might yield very different results in two different people. And as I've hinted at above in a variety of settings, it's not just a question of the medicine given to the patient, like a key fitting into a passive lock. Each of us has to figure out how the insulin works for us. As with all medications, the insulin might cause us intolerable side effects, we might not be able—because of work schedules, childcare responsibilities, or lack of organizational skills—to give ourselves the injections multiple times a day. We might not be able to afford them.

All of these details might be difficult to discuss with our primary care physician, if the relationship is not on a good footing. Yet the impulse among doctors is too often still to treat the diabetes number, the hemoglobin A1C, and not the patient.

This impulse is understandable. The large trials that have investigated effective therapies for diabetes have done so in painstakingly recruited and culled populations of thousands of people. They would be impossible to conduct if, in these trials, we tried to assess a different dose of insulin in each individual. But because the treatment must be uniform throughout the studies, their results, and the resulting recommendations by groups of doctors, only go so far.

Such professional guidelines are only now factoring in the realization that the hemoglobin A1C level of 7.0 percent, which works out to a fasting blood sugar level in the morning of 140 to 150, is not an equally effective limit for all people. In particular, recent studies have shown that so-called intensive blood sugar control, which attempts to push the hemoglobin A1C number even lower (say to 6.5, or 6 percent), can cause deleterious side effects and even increase mortality, particularly in patients with other medical problems, like heart disease.[17] Similarly, other people with fragile health conditions, like the elderly, can be harmed rather than helped if intensive glycemic control is pursued.

As with other medical decisions, there is a paucity of information. There are not multiple studies testing the effectiveness of multiple different goals for the control of blood sugar somewhere between 7 and 8 percent, two common stops on the A1C spectrum. Neither should we expect them; things can't be tuned that fine for large populations in the thousands, the size usually included in randomized clinical trials. By the same token, the doctor will never be able to tell us what particular value of blood sugar control will be best for us. There are always personally complicating factors: our reaction to insulin, our other health conditions, and things that get in the way of our adherence to treatment. In other words, execution of care processes does not depend on the patient being a machine that goes through the motions of optimizing diet and taking medicines. It depends on us as people with all our variability, and our regular doctor, with whom we have a relationship, is the one to appreciate that.

HOW TO IMPROVE COMMUNICATION IN OUR HEALTH CARE SYSTEM?

So communication with the primary care provider is important to help fix many important deficiencies with our health care system. But how do we get there? Our health system gives us one strike even before we get into the room with the doctor, because access to primary care providers is poor.[18] The Affordable Care Act, known as Obamacare, has improved coverage but has not addressed the shortage of primary care providers. Massachusetts, after providing coverage to nearly 98 percent of its citizens, has faced a shortage of primary care providers. Thus, when coverage will be extended to millions more Americans, where are they going to go to get primary care? And what kind of care will they get when they obtain access?

The two answers to this question are incentives and personalization.

Incentives: We need to pay our primary care doctors more. This of course speaks to my self-interest, since I am a primary care doctor myself. Take this obvious bias as a given, but recognize as well that the bias of specialists is even more deeply rooted in our system, and more consequential economically. While the salaries of health care professionals have declined from 1987 to 2010,[19] the salaries of medical specialists have not shared that trend, increasing compared to those of general practitioners, including primary care doctors and family practice physicians.[20]

Unsurprisingly, when medical students make decisions about their career plans, decisions that are affected by their present debt and thus their future earning potential, income difference between primary care doctors and specialists assumes great significance.[21]

Where does this salary differential come from? As I described earlier, it starts with the resource-based relative value scale, which determines how much health care providers should be paid for the services they provide. The Relative Use Committee, dominated by specialists, determines the factors by which pay is weighed. Thus, procedures that are done by those specialists are emphasized over the cognitive work, less concrete but as necessary, done by primary care and family practice doctors. As a result, the American Academy of Family Practice considered opting out of the system altogether.[22]

A revision to this system has recently been proposed as part of the Affordable Care Act.[23] This, however, is a Band-Aid on a gaping wound. The entire governing philosophy of relative value units is suspect: that medical care can be neatly broken up into individual packets. The more packets the provider delivers, the assumption goes, the better the care. But health care, we know, is not an easily measurable good. (Just look at the complications involved in measuring quality of life that I touched on in a previous chapter.) Payment to doctors should be determined by their effectiveness.

Unfortunately, this solution drags in difficulties of its own: how do we measure, exactly, the effectiveness of the medical care delivered by a physician? If mortality is the outcome of interest, we can't wait around to see whether the death rate for thirty- and forty-year-olds changes after treatment by one doctor compared to another. Perhaps we should pick the endpoints that are closely associated with certain diseases, like diabetes. Even those are not greeted by universal agreement: do we pick the hemoglobin A1C, the integrative measure of blood sugar that we have discussed in previous chapters—and if so, what level is optimal for the most people? The discussions are never ending.

The other way of providing incentives is to start with the payment, not with the services: much as hospitals have started to focus on "bundled care," trying to get as much as possible out of a given sum for each person admitted to the hospital, doctors can perhaps do the same in the outpatient setting. This focus needs to be paired, obviously, with a set of agreed-upon outcomes;

otherwise a clinic could very easily make money hand over fist by providing substandard care.

Thus we can restructure the payment system in order to guide more money to the doctors who should see us most often, the primary care providers. That term includes internal medicine doctors, pediatricians, family practice doctors, gynecologists, even psychiatrists—really everyone who sees us month in and month out, through our lifetime. And it also includes nurse practitioners and physician assistants who can also serve as primary care providers.

But paying primary care doctors more will not by itself foster relationships between us and these doctors in a way that encourages regular communication and decreases the problems we have discussed, including unchecked referrals and contraindicated testing. Here, in closing, I will make my immodest proposal, that the incentives, both for us and our doctors, as well as for hospitals, health-care systems, and medical education, need to be refocused with the doctor-patient relationship at its center.

BUILDING A NEW HEALTH CARE SYSTEM WITH RELATIONSHIPS AT THE CENTER

It is not enough to pay primary care providers more when specialists still make several times as much. Nor is it enough to encourage us to choose doctors based on publicly available quality information when that information often has little to do with what we find important in our health. We need to find a primary care provider who can be with us every step of the way through our health journey, who can build a stable relationship, so we can in turn extend that relationship to our community—and, finally, realign our health culture away from unneeded tests and technologies toward measures to preserve and improve our health.

The change will come in how we define "access to care." I believe in access, and that is why I wholeheartedly supported, with all its flaws, the Affordable Care Act. At this point, however, we should ask a further question: yes, we should improve access to health care—but access to what? Access to services that might not help, to preventive care (like mammograms and PSA tests) whose benefits are not ironclad?

We need to have access to a relationship founded on good communication. To that end, each of us should have the opportunity to choose a primary care provider who will be with us for our lifetime. We should be provided information on how well this provider communicates with his patients and be free to choose the provider on that basis. Furthermore, we and our doctors—should all be provided incentives to stick with that relationship and develop it.

What would these incentives look like and how would they work practically? Doctors could be provided a bonus for retention of their patient panel. Patients would be provided incentives to get advice, examinations, and time with their primary care provider rather than always going to specialists first. Much as employers currently provide incentives to employees for getting preventive health exams, such a culture change would encourage employers to provide incentives to employees who make a health plan with their doctor and follow up on it.

These suggestions will not be so simple to carry out. As it stands, our health care system is centered on reimbursements for procedures, and perhaps for time spent, but not for thought or building relationships. Furthermore, we are supposed to want—and many of us expect—the widest possible choice of doctors, tests, and procedures.

If incentives are recentered to encourage the development of a relationship between us and our primary care doctor, as is the case already in some integrated care organizations and as might be part of Accountable Care Organizations (though these, too, are less about doctor-patient visits than in keeping all the medical care in the same group of doctors) then it might become somewhat more difficult to obtain a full range of procedures, doctors, and tests with the immediacy we have come to expect.

IS REDUCING OVERUSE RATIONING?

Is this rationing, as health care doomsayers are wont to tell us? Yes, but in the true sense of the word "rationing," controlling access to a limited good, we all suffer now from health care rationing. Health quality is limited under the current system, and paradoxically it is parceled out unequally not just to those who don't have access to doctors, but to those who have the advantage of too many procedures. Overuse is just as much a rationing as lack of access to care; it's just that those of us who overuse, or follow the advice of doctors who overuse, do not have access to the quality care that would avoid such overuse.

If the health-care system is not providing equal quality, we should welcome a conversation with our doctor that can improve that situation by reducing overuse. On the other hand, however, we need to have a doctor with whom such conversation is welcome. That means medical schools and residencies focused on training doctors with the best communication skills, tracking those with communication talents and interest in the primary care context separately from those who would prefer to become expert in a limited set of procedures. It also means that when we talk about quality reporting, choosing the best doctors and hospitals, we should be able to choose based on outcomes that matter to a long-term patient-doctor relationship.

Research can't tell us everything yet. We know about the importance of communication but we don't know whether being told about our doctors' communication skills will, in the end, provide incentive enough to choose them or improve our health. We don't know whether emphasizing such skills in medical education will produce doctors who are better at communication.

At some point, however, as in all medical decision making, we have to make a decision based on imperfect information. Our health care system does not encourage the conversation. While starting to improve matters with our doctor, we should look out for health advocates, politicians, and hospitals that realize the importance of communication and move the health care system in the direction of improving it. We should become advocates not just for ourselves alone, but for communication-sensitive doctors and health care leaders.

Notes

1. THE MOST FREQUENT PROCEDURE

1. Judith K. Ockene, Jean Kristeller, Robert Goldberg, et al., "Increasing the efficacy of physician-delivered smoking interventions," *Journal of General Internal Medicine* 6 (1991):1–8.

2. M. Lipkin Jr., S. M. Putnam, and J. Lazare, editors. *The Medical Interview*. New York: Springer, 1994.

3. Carl Schneider. *The Practice of Autonomy: Patients, Doctors, and Medical Decisions*. New York: Oxford University Press, 1998.

2. VISIT TIME AND CLOCK TIME

1. Debra L. Roter and Judith A. Hall, *Doctors Talking With Patients/Patients Talking With Doctors: Improving Communication in Medical Visits*, Westport, CT: Greenwood Publishing, 2006.

2. D. C. Morrell, M. E. Evans, R. W. Morris, et al., "The 'five minute' consultation: Effect of time constraint on clinical content and patient satisfaction," Br Med J (Clin Res Ed) 292 (1986) DOI: http://dx.doi.org/10.1136/bmj.292.6524.870.

3. Debra L. Roter and Judith A. Hall, "Doctors Talking With Patients/Patients Talking With Doctors: Improving Communication in Medical Visits,"; Myriam Deveugele, Anselm Derese, Atie van den Brink-Muinen, et al., "Consultation length in general practice: Cross sectional study in six European countries," *BMJ* 325(2002) DOI: http://dx.doi.org/10.1136/bmj.325.7362.472.

4. H. M. Evans. "Wonder and the clinical encounter," Theor Med Bioeth (2012) 33:123–36, DOI: 10.1007/s11017-012-9214-4.

5. Lisa Cooper-Patrick, Joseph J. Gallo, and Junius J. Gonzales "Race, gender, and part-nership in the physician-patient relationship," *JAMA*. 282 (1999): 583–89. DOI:10.1001/jama.282.6.583.

6. Scott Bishop, Mark Lau, and Shauna Shapiro. "Mindfulness: A proposed operational definition," *Clinical Psychology Science and Practice* 11 (2004):230–41, DOI: 10.1093/clipsy.bph077.

7. Debra L. Roter and Judith A. Hall. *Doctors Talking With Patients/Patients Talking With Doctors*.

8. Zackary Berger, Mary Catherine Beach, et al., "Agenda-setting in routine primary HIV encounters." *Journal of General Internal Medicine* 26 (2011):S242.

9. Joanne Lynn, Janice Lynch Schuster, and Joan Harrold, *Handbook for Mortals: Guidance for People Facing Serious Illness*. New York: Oxford University Press, 2011.

3. WHAT WE WANT AS PATIENTS: LESSONS FROM COMMUNICATION SCIENCE

1. James J. Walsh, "Psychotherapy: What the modern physician thinks of the mind cure as practised in all ages," *The Independent*, September 11, 1913, p.628, http://books.google.com/books/download/The_Independent.pdf?id=6Pi0AAAAMAAJ&output=pdf&sig=ACfU3U2E0VFgf0f0o79itkYoWTho329JYg.

2. Thomas J. Beauchamp and James F. Childress, *Principles of Biomedical Ethics*. New York: Oxford University Press, 2001.

3. "U.S. Census Bureau State & Country QuickFacts, Baltimore, Maryland," accessed June 19, 2012, http://quickfacts.census.gov/qfd/states/24/24510.html.

4. R. Kaba and P. Sooniakumaran, "The evolution of the doctor-patient relationship," *International Journal of Surgery* 5 (2007): 57. http://dx.doi.org/10.1016/j.ijsu.2006.01.005

5. Michael Balint, Paul H. Ornstein, and Enid Balint, *Focal Psychotherapy*. London: Tavistock Publications, 1972, p. 76.

6. http://en.wikipedia.org/wiki/Michael_Balint, accessed June 19, 2012.

7. J. Hughes," Organization and information at the bed-side: "The Experience of the Medical Division of Labor by University Hospitals' Inpatients" (PhD diss., University of Chicago, 1994). http://www.changesurfer.com/Hlth/HuDiss.html, accessed June 19, 2012.

8. Thomas S. Szasz, William F. Knoff and Marc H. Hollender. "The doctor-patient relationship and its historical context," *Am J Psychiatry* 115 (1958):522–28.

9. Thomas S. Szasz, Marc H. Hollender. "The basic models of the doctor-patient relationship," *Archives of Internal Medicine* 97 (1956):585.

10. D. L. Roter, M. Stewart, S. M. Putnam, M. Lipkin Jr., W. Stiles, and T. S. Inui. "Communication patterns of primary care physicians," *JAMA* 277 (1997):350–56.

11. R. Adams, K. Price, G. Tucker, A. M. Nguyen, D. Wilson, "The doctor and the patient—how is a clinical encounter perceived?" *Patient Education and Counseling* 86 (2012):127–33.

12. Debra Roter and Judith A. Hall. *Doctors Talking to Patients/Patients Talking to Doctors*. Westport, CT: Greenwood Publishing Group, 2006.

13. L. A. Cooper, D. Roter, R. Johnson et al. "Patient-centered communication, ratings of care, and concordance of patient and physician race," *Annals of Internal Medicine* 139 (2003):907–15.

14. L. A. Cooper, D. L. Roter, K. A. Carson et al., "The associations of clinicians' implicit attitudes about race with medical visit communication and patient ratings of interpersonal care," *American Journal of Public Health* 102 (2012):979–87.

15. Jerome Groopman, *How Doctors Think*. New York: Houghton Mifflin Harcourt, 2007.

16. R. J. Ablin, "Invited commentary—prostate cancer: Doing less might be more," *Archives of Internal Medicine* 170(2010):1397–99.

17. C. Hofmann, N. S. Wenger, R. B. Davis, et al. "Patient preferences for communication with physicians about end-of-life decisions," *Annals of Internal Medicine* 127 (1997):1–12.

18. S. E. Inzucchi, R. M. Bergenstal, J. B. Buse, et al. "Management of hyperglycemia in type 2 diabetes: A patient centered approach: Position Statement of the American Diabetes Association (ADA) and the European Association for the Study of Diabetes (EASD)," *Diabetes Care* 35 (2012):1364–79.

19. A. A. Montgomery, J. Harding, T. Fahey, "Shared decision making in hypertension: the impact of patient preferences on treatment choice," *Family Practice* 18 (2001):309–13.

20. David B. Reuben and Mary E. Tinetti, "Goal-Oriented patient care—an alternative health outcomes paradigm," *New England Journal of Medicine* 366 (2012):777–79

21. W. M. Strull, B. Lo, G. Charles, "Do patients want to participate in medical decision making?" *Journal of the American Medical Association* 252 (1984):2990–94.

22. Debra Roter and Judith A. Hall. *Doctors Talking to Patients/Patients Talking to Doctors*. Westport, CT: Greenwood Publishing Group, 2006, p. xx.

4. THE DOCTOR AS A PROFESSIONAL—IN OUR EYES

1. Atul Gawande, *Complications*. New York: Metropolitan Books, 2002.

2. David Barnard, "The physician as priest, revisited," *Journal of Religion and Health* 24 (1985): 272–286, DOI: 10.1007/BF01533009.

3. M. Yin, S. Bastacky, U. Chandran, M. J. Becich, and R. Dhir, "Prevalence of incidental prostate cancer in the general population: A study of healthy organ donors," *Journal Urology* 179 (2008):892–95.

4. http://www.uspreventiveservicestaskforce.org/uspstf/uspsbrca.htm. Accessed July 1, 2012.

5. N. Calonge, D. B. Petitti, T. G. DeWitt, et al., "Screening for breast cancer: U.S. Preventive Services Task Force recommendation statement," *Annals of Internal Medicine* 151 (2009):716-26.

6. M. L. Gourlay, J. P. Fine, J. S. Preisser, et al., Study of Osteoporotic Fractures Research Group, "Bone-density testing interval and transition to osteoporosis in older women," *New England Journal of Medicine* 366 (2012):225–33.

7. http://en.wikipedia.org/wiki/Hippocratic_Oath. Accessed July 1, 2012.

8. Eric Campbell, Susan Regan, Russell Gruen, et al., "Professionalism in medicine: Results of a national survey of physicians," *Annals Of Internal Medicine* 147 (2007):795-W234.

9. P. Wagner, J. Hendrich, G. Moseley, and V. Hudson, "Defining medical professionalism: A qualitative study," *Medical Education* 41 (2007):288–94.

10. Donald A. Misch, "Evaluating physicians' professionalism and humanism: The case for humanism 'connoisseurs,'" *Academic Medicine* 77 (2002):489–95.

11. http://www.iom.edu/Reports/2012/Primary-Care-and-Public-Health.aspx. Accessed July1, 2012.

12. Pauline W. Chen, "Can Doctors Learn Empathy," *New York Times* Well blog, June 21, 2012, http://well.blogs.nytimes.com/2012/06/21/can-doctors-learn-empathy/. Accessed July 1, 2012.

13. http://videos.howstuffworks.com/university-of-florida/21812-teaching-doctors-to-recognize-racism-video.htm. Accessed July 1, 2012.

14. Ludwig Edelstein, "The Hippocratic Oath: Text, Translation, and Interpretation," Baltimore: The Johns Hopkins University Press, 1964, 64.

5. MEASURING HOW GOOD OUR DOCTORS ARE

1. Atul Gawande, *The Checklist Manifesto: How to Get Things Right*. New York: Profile Books, 2010.

2. Peter Pronovost, Eric Vohr, *Safe Patients, Smart Hospitals: How One Doctor's Checklist Can Help Change Healthcare From the Inside Out*. New York: Penguin, 2010.

3. Peter M. Fayers and David Machin, *Quality of Life: The Assessment, Analysis, and Interpretation of Patient-Reported Outcomes*, New York: John Wiley & Sons, 2007.

4. http://www.consumerreports.org/cro/magazine/2012/08/how-safe-is-your-hospital/index.htm. Accessed July 14, 2012.

5. http://www.hospitalcompare.hhs.gov/hospital-search.aspx? AspxAutoDetectCookieSupport=1. Accessed July 14, 2012.

6. E. Morsi, P. K. Lindenauer, M. B. Rothberg, "Primary care physicians' use of publicly reported quality data in hospital referral decisions," *Journal of Hospital Medicine* 7(2012): 370–75, DOI: 10.1002/jhm.1931

7. http://health.usnews.com/best-hospitals. Accessed July 14, 2012.

8. http://health.usnews.com/health-news/best-hospitals/articles/2011/07/18/best-hospitals-2011-12-the-methodology. Accessed July 14, 2012.

9. Ashwini Sehgal, "The role of reputation in *U.S News & World Report*'s rankings of the top 50 American hospitals," *Annals of Internal Medicine* 152(2010):521–25.

10. I. B. DeGroot, W. Otten, H. J. Smeets. et al., "Is the impact of hospital performance data greater in patients who have compared hospitals?" *BMC Health Services Research* 11(2011): 214.

11. Harold S. Luft, Deborah W. Garnick, David H. Mark, et al., "Does Quality Influence Choice of Hospital?" *Journal of the American Medical Association* 263(1990):2899-2906. DOI:10.1001/jama.1990.03440210049031.

12. http://www.hcahpsonline.org/home.aspx. Accessed July 12, 2012.

13. http://www.hcahpsonline.org/files/HCAHPS%20Survey%20Results%20Table%20(Report_ HEI_October_2011_States).pdf. Accessed July 12, 2012.

14. M. Laakso, H. Cederberg, "Glucose control in diabetes: Which target level to aim for?" *Journal of Internal Medicine* 272(2012):1–12. DOI:10.1111/j.1365-2796.2012.02528.x

15. Peter Pronovost, Eric Vohr, *Safe Patients, Smart Hospitals: How One Doctor's Checklist Can Help Change Healthcare From the Inside Out*. New York: Penguin, 2010.

16. A. Jerant, P. Franks, and R. L. Kravitz, "Associations between pain control self-efficacy, self-efficacy for communicating with physicians, and subsequent pain severity among cancer patients," *Patient Educ Couns*. 85(2011):275–80.

17. http://www.cms.gov/Medicare/Quality-Initiatives-Patient-Assessment-Instruments/hospital-value-based-purchasing/index.html?redirect=/Hospital-Value-Based-Purchasing/. Accessed July 12, 2012.

18. Gretchen M. Ray, James J. Nawarskas, and Joe R. Anderson, "Blood pressure monitoring technique impacts hypertension treatment," *Journal of General Internal Medicine* 27(2012):623-629. DOI: 10.1007/s11606-011-1937-9.

19. S. V. Srinivas, R. A. Deyo, Z.D. Berger, "Application of less is more to low back pain." *Archives of Internal Medicine* 2012: Jun 4, 1–5. DOI: 10.1001/archinternmed.2012.1838

6. TELLING OUR STORY: TAKING THE TIME TO EXPRESS OUR HEALTH CONCERNS TO OURSELVES AND OTHERS

1. http://www.cdc.gov/nchs/data/series/sr_10/sr10_252.pdf. Accessed July 30, 2012.

2. Rita Charon, "Narrative and medicine," *New England Journal of Medicine* 350(2004):862–4.

3. Christine Laine, "The annual physical examination: Needless ritual or necessary routine?" *Annals of Internal Medicine* 136(202):701–3.

4. Linei Urban and Cicero Urban, "Role of mammography versus magnetic resonance imaging for breast cancer screening," *Current Breast Cancer Reports* 2012, http://dx.doi.org/10.1007/s12609-012-0085-5.

5. http://www.uspreventiveservicestaskforce.org/uspstf/uspscerv.htm. Accessed July 30, 2012.

6. http://www.uspreventiveservicestaskforce.org/uspstf/uspschol.htm. Accessed July 30, 2012.

7. S. H. Wolff and R. Harris, "The harms of testing: New attention to an old concern," *Journal of the American Medical Association*, 307(2012):565–66.

7. MAKE THE MOST OF THE VISIT THROUGH MINDFULNESS

1. Gardner Harris, "New for aspiring doctors, the people skills test," *New York Times*, July 10, 2011;M. Deveugele, et al. "Teaching communication skills to medical students, a challenge in the curriculum?" *Patient Education and Counseling* 58 (2005):265–70.

2. D. C. Chen et al., "Characterizing changes in student empathy throughout medical school." *Medical Teaching* 34 (2012):305–11.

3. Robert M. Anderson and Martha M. Funnell, "Negotiating behavioral changes with patients who have diabetes: Negotiation or coercion?" *Diabetes Management* 2 (2012):41–46.

4. Diane R. Rittenhouse, "The patient centered medical home: Will it stand the test of health reform?" *JAMA* 301 (2009):2038–40.

5. R. S. Beck, R. Daughtridge and P. D. Sloane, "Physician-patient communication in the primary care office: A systematic review," *J Am Board Fam Pract* 15 (2002):25–38.

6. H. B. Beckman, R. A. Frankel, "The effect of physician behavior on the collection of data," *Annals of Internal Medicine* 101 (1984):692–96.

7. L. A. Hanyok et al., "Practicing patient-centered care: The questions clinically excellent physicians use to get to know their patients as individuals," *The Patient* 5 (2012):141–45.

8. http://www.slideshare.net/samueljack/466-enhancing-communication-and-hiv-outcomes-the-echo-studyppt. Accessed August 12, 2012.

9. I. Hsu et al, "Providing support to patients in emotional encounters: A new perspective on missed empathic opportunities," *Patient Education and Counseling* 2012 Jul 17.

10. Paul Rosseau, "Empathy," *Journal of Hospital and Palliative Care* 25 (2008):261–62, DOI: 10.1177/1049909108315524AM.

11. A. L. Suchman and D. A. Matthews, "What makes the patient-doctor relationship therapeutic? Exploring the connexional dimension of medical care," *Ann Intern Med* 108 (1988):125

12. C. Bieber et al., "Training physicians in shared decision making: Who can be reached and what is achieved?" *Patient Education and Counseling* 77 (2009):48–54.

13. I. Hsu et al., "Providing support to patients in emotional encounters: A new perspective on missed empathic opportunities," *Patient Education and Counseling* 2012 Jul 17.

8. HOW TO COMMUNICATE EVEN WHILE INTIMIDATED, LIMITED, UNCOMFORTABLE, OR UNDEREDUCATED

1. http://en.wikipedia.org/wiki/Internet_in_the_United_States.

2. Zackary Berger, Anne Dembitzer, and Mary Catherine Beach, "Reason for hospital admission: A pilot study comparing patient statements to chart reports." *Narrative Inquiry in Bioethics*, in press.

3. Marjorie Kagawa-Singer and Shaheen Kassim-Lakha, "A strategy to reduce cross-cultural miscommunication and increase the likelihood of improving health outcomes," *Academic Medicine* 78 (2003):577–87.

4. D. Diao, J. M. Wright, D. K. Cundiff, et al., "Pharmacotherapy for mild hypertension," *Cochrane Database Syst Rev* 8(2012):CD006742.

5. Otis W. Brawley, "Prostate cancer screening: What we know, don't know, and believe," *Ann Intern Med.* 157(2012):135–36.

6. W. Morrison, "Is that all you got?" J Palliat Med 13(2010):1384–85.

7. F. Sparrenberger, F. T., Cichelero, A. M. Fonseca, et al., "Does psychosocial stress cause hypertension? A systematic review of observational studies," *J Hum Hypertens* 23(2009):12–19.

8. Myfanwy Morgan, C. J. Watkins, "Managing hypertension: Beliefs and responses to medication among cultural groups," *Sociology of Health & Illness* 10(1998):561–78.

9. Barbara A. Israel et al., "Review of community-based research: Assessing partnership-based approaches to improve public health," *Annual Review of Public Health* 19 (1998):173–202.

10. Judith Belle Brown, W. Wayne Weston, and Moira A. Stewart, "Patient-Centred interviewing part II: finding common ground," *Can Fam Physician* 35(1989): 153–57.

11. http://zocalopublicsquare.org/thepublicsquare/2011/11/30/how-doctors-die/read/nexus/. Accessed October 22, 2012.

12. Diao D, Wright J.M., Cundiff D.K., Gueyffier F. Pharmacotherapy for mild hypertension. Cochrane Database Syst Rev. 2012 Aug 15;8:CD006742. doi: 10.1002/14651858.CD006742.pub2.

13. Dominick Frosch, Suepattra May, Katharine Rendle, et al., "Authoritarian physicians and patients' fear of being labeled 'difficult' among key obstacles to shared decision making," *Health Affairs* 31(2012):1030–38.

14. Tom L. Delbanco, "Enriching the doctor-patient relationship by inviting the patient's perspective," *Ann Intern Med.* 116(1992):414–18.

9. WHAT WE'RE TALKING ABOUT: NEGOTIATING THE AGENDA WITH THE DOCTOR

1. K. Dwan, D. G. Altman, J. A. Arnaiz, et al., "Systematic review of the empirical evidence of study publication bias and outcome reported bias," *PLoS ONE* 3(2008):e3081. DOI:10.1371/journal.pone.0003081.

2. D. Diao, J. M. Wright, D. K. Cundiff, et al., "Pharmacotherapy for mild hypertension," Cochrane Database System Reviews 8(2012):CD006742.

3. L. Blonde, "Benefits and risks for intensive glycemic control in patients with diabetes mellitus," *American Journal of the Medical Sciences* 343(2012):17–20

4. M. K. Marvel, R. M. Epstein, K. Flowers, et al., "Soliciting the patient's agenda: have we improved?" *JAMA* 281(1999):283–87.

5. J. L. Jackson and K. Kroenke, "The effect of unmet expectations among adults presenting with physical symptoms," *Annals of Internal Medicine* 134(2001):889–97.

6. D. M. Brock, L. B. Mauksch, S. Witteborn, et al., "Effectiveness of intensive physician training in upfront agenda setting," *Journal of General Internal Medicine* 26(2011):1317–23.

7. Richard J. Botelho, "A negotiation model for the doctor-patient relationship," *Family Practice* 9 (1992) : 210–18. DOI: 10.1093/fampra/9.2.210.

8. R. L. Kravitz, R. A. Bell, and C. E. Franz, " A taxonomy of requests by patients (TORP): A new system for understanding clinical negotiation in office practice," *Journal of Family Practice* 48(1999):872–78.

9. S.V. Srinivas, R.A. Deyo, and Z.D. Berger, "Application of "less is more" to low back pain," *Arch Intern Med* 172(2012):1016–20.

10. W. C. Jacobs, M. P. Arts, M. W. van Tulder, et al., "Surgical techniques for sciatica due to herniated disc, a systematic review," *European Spine Journal* July 20, 2012.

10. ACKNOWLEDGE — AND USE — EMOTION AND MOTIVATION

1. Jerome Groopman, *How Doctors Think*. New York: Houghton Mifflin, 2007.

2. Carl R. Rogers, "The necessary and sufficient conditions of therapeutic personality change," *Journal of Consulting Psychiatry* 21(1957):95–103.

3. Jerome Groopman, *How Doctors Think*.

4. Gordana Stevanovic, Gordana Tucakovic, Rajko Dotlic, and Vladimir Kanjuh, "Correlation of clinical diagnoses with autopsy findings: A retrospective study of 2,145 consecutive autopsies," *Human Pathology* 17(1986):1225–30.

5. Antonio Damasio, *Descartes' Error: Emotion, Reason and the Human Brain*. New York: Random House, 2008.

6. William R. Miller and Steven P. Rollnick, *Motivational Interviewing, Preparing People for Change*. New York: Guilford Press, 2002.

7. S. Rubak, A. Sandbaek, T. Lauritzen, and B. Christensen, "Motivational interviewing: A systematic review and meta-analysis," *B J Gen Pract*. 55(2005):305–12.

8. F. M. Walter, J. Emery, "Perceptions of family history across common diseases: A qualitative study in primary care," *Fam Pract* 23(2006):472–80.

9. Mandy Ryan and Shelley Farrar, "Using conjoint analysis to elicit preferences for health care," *British Medical Journal* 320(2000):1530–33.

10. H. M. Warwick and P. M. Salkovskis, "Reassurance," *British Medical Journal* (Clinical Research Edition), 290(1985): 1028.

11. Brett D. Thombs, James C. Coyne, Pim Cuijpers, et al., "Rethinking recommendations for screening for depression in primary care," *CMAJ* 184(2012):413–18.

12. Margaret S. Chisolm and Constantine G. Lyketsos, *Systematic Psychiatric Evaluation*. Baltimore: Johns Hopkins University Press, 2012.

13. Michael J. Barry and Susan Edgman-Levitan, "Shared decision making—the pinnacle of patient-centered care," *New England Journal of Medicine* 366(2012):780–81.

11. HOW TO TALK TO THE DOCTOR ABOUT WHAT MAKES YOU NERVOUS, EMBARRASSED, OR GROSSED OUT

1. D. L. Roter and J. A. Hall, "Physician gender and patient-centered communication: A critical review of empirical research," *Annu Rev Public Health* 25(2004):497–519.

2. Zackary Berger, Anne Dembitzer, and Mary Catherine Beach, "Reason for hospital admission: A pilot study comparing patient statements to chart reports." *Narrative Inquiry in Bioethics*, in press.

3. W.E. Whitehead, " Diagnosing and managing fecal incontinence: If you don't ask, they won't tell," *Gastroenterology* 129(2005):6.]

4. N. Haley, B. Maheux, M. Rivard, et al., "Sexual health risk assessment and counseling in primary care: How involved are general practitioners and obstetrician-gynecologists?" *Am J Public Health*. 89(1999):899– 902.

5. S. Read, M. King, and J Watson, "Sexual dysfunction in primary medical care: Prevalence, characteristics and detection by the general practitioner," *J Public Health Med*. 19(1997):387– 91.

6. Sherwin Nuland, *How We Die: Reflections on Life's Final Chapter*. New York: Random House, 2000.

7. E. K. Fromme, D. Zive, T. A. Schmidt, et al., "POLST Registry do-not-resuscitate orders and other patient treatment preferences." *JAMA*. 307(2012):34–35.

8. J. K. Yuen, M. C. Reid, and M. D. Fetters, "Hospital do-not-resuscitate orders: Why they have failed and how to fix them," *J Gen Intern Med*. 26(2011):79–7.

9. E. K. Vig, H. Starks, J. S. Taylor, et al., "Surviving surrogate decision-making: What helps and hampers the experience of making medical decisions for others," *J Gen Intern Med*. 2(2007):1274–79.

10. D. P. Sulmasy and L. Snyder, "Substituted interests and best judgments: An integrated model of surrogate decision making," *JAMA* 304(2010):1946–7.

11. E. A. Rider, M. M. Hinrichs, and B. A. Lown, "A model for communication skills assessment across the undergraduate curriculum," Med Teach 28(2006):127–34; H. M. Bosse, M. Nickel, S. Huwendiek et al., "Peer role-play and standardised patients in communication training: A comparative study on the student perspective on acceptability, realism, and perceived effect," *BMC Med Educ* 10(2010):27.

12. MAKING HEALTHY COMMUNITIES WITH HEALTHY COMMUNICATION

1. A. Vastine, J. Gittelsohn, B. Ethelbah, et al., "Formative research and stakeholder participation in intervention development," *Am J Health Behav* 29(2005):57–69.

2. Namratha R. Kandula, Neerja R. Khurana, Gregory Makoul, et al., "A community and culture-centered approach to developing effective cardiovascular health messages," *Journal of General Internal Medicine* 27(2012):1308–16.

3. Michael Osterholme, Nicholas Kelley, Alfred Sommer, et al., "Efficacy and effectiveness of influenza vaccines: A systematic review and meta-analysis," *Lancet Infectious Diseases* 12(2011):36–44.

4. Arthur Caplan, "Quantifying the efficacy of influenza vaccines," *Lancet Infectious Diseases* 12(2012):656–57.

5. Karen G. Wooten, Pascale M. Wortley, James A. Singleton, et al., "Perceptions matter: Beliefs about influenza vaccine and vaccination behavior among elderly white, black and Hispanic Americans," *Vaccine* 30(2012):6927–34.

6. Rebecca Skloot, *The Immortal Life of Henrietta Lacks*. New York: Macmillan, 2010.

7. R. J. Wray, K. Jupka, W. Ross, et al., "How can you improve vaccination rates among older African Americans?" *J Fam Pract*, 56 (2007):925–29.

8. Steven Woloshin and Lisa M. Schwartz, "How a charity oversells mammography," *British Medical Journal* 2012; 345.

9. Comilla Sasson, David J. Magid, Paul Chan, et al., "Association of neighborhood characteristics with bystander-initiated CPR," *New England Journal of Medicine* 367(2012):1607–15.

10. http://www.nytimes.com/2012/09/14/nyregion/health-board-votes-to-regulate-jewish-circumcision-ritual.html. Accessed November 23, 2012.

11. http://www.thehastingscenter.org/Bioethicsforum/Post.aspx?id=5959&blogid=140. Accessed November 23, 2012.

12. R.S. Taylor et al. Reduced Dietary Salt for the Prevention of Cardiovascular Disease: A Meta-Analysis of Randomized Controlled Trials (Cochrane Review). *Am J Hypertens* (2011) 24 (8): 843-853. Doi: 10.1038/ajh.2011.115

13. http://www.cdc.gov/diabetes/statistics/prev/national/figbyage.htm. Accessed November 23, 2012.

14. C. T. Thorpe, L. E. Fahey, and H. Johnson, "Facilitating healthy coping in patients with diabetes: A systematic review," Diabetes Educ October 16, 2012. doi: 10.1177/0145721712464400.

15. Laurie Ruggiero, Amparo Castillo, Lauretta Quinn and Michelle Hochwert, "Translation of the Diabetes Prevention Program's Lifestyle Intervention: Role of community health workers," *Current Diabetes Reports* 2012, 12:127–37. DOI: 10.1007/s11892-012-0254-y.

16. F. Glans, K. F. Eriksson, A. Segerström, et al., "Evaluation of the effects of exercise on insulin sensitivity in Arabian and Swedish women with type 2 diabetes," *Diabetes Res Clin Pract* 85(2009):69–74.

17. P. A. Singer, E. S. Tasch, C. Stocking, et al., "Sex or survival: Trade-offs between quality and quantity of life." *J Clin Oncol* 9(1991):328–34.

13. LEARNING HOW TO WANT LESS: CREATING A RESOURCE-SPARING MEDICAL CULTURE TOGETHER WITH OUR DOCTORS

1. Jerome Groopman and Pamela Hartzband, *Your Medical Mind: How to Decide What is Right for You.* New York: Penguin Press, 2011.

2. Timothy J. Wilt, Michael K. Brawer, Karen M. Jones, et al., for the PIVOT Study Group. "Radical prostatectomy versus observation for localized prostate cancer," *New England Journal of Medicine* 367(2012):203–13. DOI: 10.1056/NEJMoa1113162.

3. Virginia A. Moyer, "Screening for prostate cancer: U.S. Preventive Services Task Force Recommendation Statement," *Annals of Internal Medicine* 157(2012):120–34.

4. Robert A. Smith, Vilma Cokkinides, Durado Brooks, et al., "Cancer screening in the United States, 2010: A review of current American Cancer Society guidelines and issues in cancer screening," *CA* 60(2010). DOI: 10.3322/caac.20063.

5. Christine K. Cassel and James A. Guest, "Choosing wisely: Helping physicians and patients make smart decisions about their care," *Journal of the American Medical Association* 307(2012):1801–02. DOI:10.1001/jama.2012.476.

6. S. V. Srinivas, R. A. Deyo, Z. D. Berger, "Application of 'less is more' to low back pain," *Archives of Internal Medicine* 172(2012):1016–20. doi:10.1001/archintern-med.2012.1838.

7. Jeanne Lenzer, "Cochrane review finds no proved benefit in drug treatment for patients with mild hypertension," *BMJ* 2012:345. DOI: http://dx.doi.org/10.1136/bmj.e5511

8. Jan Walker, Immy Holloway, and Beatrice Sofaer, "In the system: The lived experience of chronic back pain from the perspectives of those seeking help from pain clinics," *Pain* 80(1999):621–28, http://dx.doi.org/10.1016/S0304-3959(98)00254-1.

9. Jane C. Weeks, Paul J. Catalano, Angel Cronin, et al., "Patients' expectations about effects of chemotherapy for advanced cancer," *N Engl J Med* 367(2012):1616–25. DOI: 10.1056/NEJMoa1204410.

10. Gregory L. Armstrong, Laura A. Conn, and Robert W. Pinner, "Trends in infectious disease mortality in the United States during the 20th century," *JAMA.* 281(1999):61–66. DOI:10-1001/pubs.JAMA-ISSN-0098-7484-281-1-joc80862.

11. Elizabeth G. Nabel and Eugene Braunwald, "A tale of coronary artery disease and myocardial infarction," *N Engl J Med* 366(2012):54–63. DOI: 10.1056/NEJMra1112570.

12. Roger Detels, Alvaro Muñoz, Glen McFarlane, et al., for the Multicenter AIDS Cohort Study Investigators, "Effectiveness of potent antiretroviral therapy on time to AIDS and death in men with known HIV infection duration," *JAMA.* 280(1998):1497–1503. DOI:10-

13. Madhukar H. Trivedi, A. John Rush, Stephen R. Wisniewski, et al., for the STAR*D Study Team, "Evaluation of outcomes with Citalopram for depression using measurement-based care in STAR*D: Implications for clinical practice," *Am J Psychiatry* 163(2006):28–40.DOI:10.1176/appi.ajp.163.1.28.

14. S. Hughes, D. Cohen, "A systematic review of long-term studies of drug treated and non-drug treated depression," *J Affect Disord.* 118(2009):9–18.

15. Cathy Schoen, Robin Osborn, Michelle M. Doty, et al., "Toward Higher-Performance Health Systems: Adults' Health Care Experiences In Seven Countries, 2007," *Health Aff* 26(2007):w717–w734, DOI: 10.1377/hlthaff.26.6.w717.

16. Donald M. Berwick, Andrew D. Hackbarth, "Eliminating waste in US health care," *JAMA.* 307(2012):1513–16. DOI:10.1001/jama.2012.362.

17. Daniel Kahneman, "A different approach to health state valuation," *Value in Health* 12(2009):516–17.

18. Elliot Fisher, David Wennberg, Therese Stukel, et al., "The implications of regional variations in Medicare spending, part 1: The content, quality, and accessibility of care, *Annals of Internal Medicine* 138(2003):273–87.

19. K. E. Joynt, E. J. Orav, A. K. Jha, "The association between hospital volume and processes, outcomes, and costs of care for congestive heart failure," Ann Intern Med. 154(2011): 94–102, DOI: 10.1059/0003-4819-154-2-201101180-00008.

20. R. S. Stafford, "Off-Label use of drugs and medical devices: A review of policy implications," *Clinical Pharmacology & Therapeutics* (2012); advance online publication April 4, 2012. DOI:10.1038/clpt.2012.22.

21. Judith R. McNamara, G. Russell Warnick, and Gerald R. Cooper, "A brief history of lipid and lipoprotein measurements and their contribution to clinical chemistry," *Clinica Chimica Acta* 369(2006):158–67.

22. Good Stewardship Working Group, "The Top 5 lists in primary care: Meeting the responsibility of professionalism," *Archives of Internal Medicine* 171(2011):1385.

23. Amir Qaseem, Patrick Alguire, Paul Dallas, et al., "Appropriate use of screening and diagnostic tests to foster high-value, cost-conscious care," Ann Intern Med. 156(2012):147–49.

14. TRANSFORMING OUR HEALTH CARE SYSTEM THROUGH COMMUNICATION AND COLLABORATION

1. Dave DeBronkart, "Gimme my damn data," presentation at Medicine 2.0, 2009. At http://www.slideshare.net/ePatientDave/gimme-my-damn-data-epatient-daves-keynote-at-medicine-20-2009. Accessed on December 3, 2012.

2. Tom Delbanco, Donald M. Berwick, and Jo Ivey Boufford, "Healthcare in a land called PeoplePower: Nothing about me without me," *Health Expectations* 4(2001):144–50. DOI: 10.1046/j.1369-6513.2001.00145.x.

3. W. Levinson, A. Kao, A. Kuby, et al., "Not all patients want to participate in decision making: A national study of public preferences," J Gen Intern Med 20(2005):531–5. DOI: 10.1111/j.1525-1497.2005.04101.x.

4. S. Joffe, M. Manocchia, J. C. Weeks, et al., "What do patients value in their hospital care? An empirical perspective on autonomy centred bioethics," *J Med Ethics* 29(2003):103–8.

5. http://www.cms.gov/About-CMS/Agency-Information/EEOInfo/Downloads/Annual-LanguageAccessAssessmentOutcomeReport.pdf. Accessed December 3, 2012.

6. Howard Rusk and Jason Novey, "The effect of chronic illness on families," *Marriage and Family Living* 1957;193–97.

7. Donald M. Berwick and Andrew D. Hackbarth, "Eliminating waste in US health care," *JAMA*. 307(2012):1513–16. DOI:10.1001/jama.2012.362.

8. Eric E. Fortess and Marshall B. Kapp, "medical uncertainty, diagnostic testing, and legal liability," *The Journal of Law, Medicine & Ethics* 13(1985):213–18. DOI: 10.1111/j.1748-720X.1985.tb00925.x.

9. Ronald M. Epstein, Peter Franks, and Cleveland G. Shields, "Patient-Centered Communication and Diagnostic Testing," Ann Fam Med 3(2005):415–21. DOI: 10.1370/afm.348

10. H. D. Nelson, K. Tyne, A. Naik, "Screening for breast cancer: Systematic evidence review update for the US Preventive Services Task Force," *Ann Intern Med.* 151(2009): 727–W242. DOI: 10.1059/0003-4819-151-10-200911170-00009.

11. Archie Bleyer AND H. Gilbert Welch, "Effect of three decades of screening mammography on breast-cancer incidence," *N Engl J Med* 367(2012):1998–2005. DOI: 10.1056/NEJMoa1206809.

12. http://www.cancer.gov/bcrisktool/. Accessed December 3, 2012.

13. Peter Pronovost and Eric Vohr, *Safe Patients, Smart Hospitals.* New York: Hudson Street Press, 2010.

14. Martin Makary, *Unaccountable: What Hospitals Won't Tell You and How Transparency Can Revolutionize Health Care.* New York: Bloomsbury Press, 2012.

15. S. Bolen, L. Feldman, J. Vassy, et al., "Systematic review: Comparative effectiveness and safety of oral medications for type 2 diabetes mellitus," Ann Intern Med. 147(2007):386–99.

16. Wendy Bennett, Nisa Maruthur, Sonal Singh, et al., "Comparative effectiveness and safety of medications for type 2 diabetes: An update including new drugs and 2-drug combinations," Ann Intern Med. 154(2011):602–13.

17. The Action to Control Cardiovascular Risk in Diabetes Study Group. "Effects of intensive glucose lowering in type 2 diabetes," *N Engl J Med* 358(2008):2545–59. DOI: 10.1056/NEJMoa0802743.

18. Phuong Trang Huynh, Cathy Schoen, Robin Osborn, et al., "The U.S. health care divide: Disparities in primary care experiences by income," (2006) The Commonwealth Fund. http://www.commonwealthfund.org/Publications/Fund-Reports/2006/Apr/The-U-S-Health-Care-Divide-Disparities-in-Primary-Care-Experiences-by-Income.aspx. Accessed December 4, 2012.

19. Seth A. Seabury, Anupam B. Jena, and Amitabh Chandra, "Trends in the earnings of health care professionals in the United States, 1987–2010," *JAMA*. 308(2012):2083–85. DOI:10.1001/jama.2012.14552.

20. G. C. Pope, J. E. Schneider, "Trends in physician income," *Health Affairs* 11(1992):181–93. DOI: 10.1377/hlthaff.11.1.181.

21. Martha S. Grayson, Dale A. Newton, and Lori F. Thompson, "Payback time: The associations of debt and income with medical student career choice," Medical Education 46(2012):983–91. DOI: 10.1111/j.1365-2923.2012.04340.x.

22. James Arvantes, "Delegates send message to AAFP leaders: Withdraw from the RUC," *AAFP News Now*, May 11, 2011. http://www.aafp.org/online/en/home/publications/news/news-now/inside-aafp/20110511ncscruc.html. Accessed December 4, 2012.

23. "Medicare Program; Revisions to Payment Policies Under the Physician Fee Schedule, DME Face-to-Face Encounters, Elimination of the Requirement for Termination of Non-Random Prepayment Complex Medical Review and Other Revisions to Part B for CY 2013," Federal Register 77(2012): 68891-69373. http://www.gpo.gov/fdsys/pkg/FR-2012-11-16/pdf/2012-26900.pdf. Accessed December 4, 2012.

Bibliography

Ablin, R. J. "Invited commentary—prostate cancer: doing less might be more," *Archives of Internal Medicine* 170(2010):1397–99.

The Action to Control Cardiovascular Risk in Diabetes Study Group. "Effects of intensive glucose lowering in type 2 diabetes," *N Engl J Med* 358(2008):2545–59. DOI: 10.1056/NEJMoa0802743.

Adams, R., K. Price, G. Tucker, A. M. Nguyen, and D. Wilson. "The doctor and the patient—how is a clinical encounter perceived?," *Patient Education and Counseling* 86 (2012):127–33.

Anderson, Robert M. and Martha M. Funnell. "Negotiating behavioral changes with patients who have diabetes: negotiation or coercion?" *Diabetes Management* 2 (2012):41–46.

Armstrong, Gregory L., Laura A. Conn, and Robert W. Pinner. "Trends in infectious disease mortality in the United States during the 20th century," *JAMA.* 281(1999):61–66. DOI:10-1001/pubs.JAMA-ISSN-0098-7484-281-1-joc80862.

Arvantes, James. "Delegates Send Message to AAFP Leaders: Withdraw From the RUC," *AAFP News Now*, May 11, 2011. http://www.aafp.org/online/en/home/publications/news/news-now/inside-aafp/20110511ncscruc.html. Accessed December 4, 2012.

Balint, Michael, Paul H. Ornstein, and Enid Balint. *Focal Psychotherapy.* London: Tavistock Publications, 1972.

Barnard, David. "The physician as priest, revisited," *Journal of Religion and Health* 24 (1985): 272–286, DOI: 10.1007/BF01533009.

Barry. Michael J. and Susan Edgman-Levitan. "Shared Decision Making—The pinnacle of patient-centered care." *New England Journal of Medicine* 366(2012):780–81.

Beauchamp, Thomas J. and James F. Childress. *Principles of Biomedical Ethics.* New York: Oxford University Press, 2001.

Beck, R. S., R. Daughtridge, and P. D. Sloane. "Physician-patient communication in the primary care office: a systematic review," *J Am Board Fam Pract* 15 (2002):25–38.

Beckman, H. B. and R. A. Frankel. "The effect of physician behavior on the collection of data," *Annals of Internal Medicine* 101 (1984):692–96.

Bennett, Wendy, Nisa Maruthur, Sonal Singh, et al. "Comparative effectiveness and safety of medications for type 2 diabetes: An update including new drugs and 2-drug combinations," *Annals of Internal Medicine* 154(2011):602–613.

Berger, Zackary, Anne Dembitzer, and Mary Catherine Beach. "Reason for hospital admission: a pilot study comparing patient statements to chart reports." *Narrative Inquiry in Bioethics*, in press.

Berger, Zackary, and Mary Catherine Beach, et al. Agenda-setting in routine primary HIV encounters. *Journal of General Internal Medicine* 26 (2011):S242.

Berwick, Donald M., Andrew D. Hackbarth, "Eliminating waste in US health care," *JAMA*. 307(2012):1513–1516. DOI:10.1001/jama.2012.362.

Bieber C., et al. "Training physicians in shared decision making: who can be reached and what is achieved?" *Patient Education and Counseling* 77 (2009):48–54.

Bishop, Scott, Mark Lau, and Shauna Shapiro. "Mindfulness: A Proposed Operational Definition," *Clinical Psychology Science and Practice* 11(2004):230–241, DOI: 10.1093/clipsy.bph077.

Bleyer, Archie, and H. Gilbert Welch. "Effect of Three Decades of Screening Mammography on Breast-Cancer Incidence," *N Engl J Med* 367(2012):1998–2005. DOI: 10.1056/NEJMoa1206809.

Blonde, L. "Benefits and risks for intensive glycemic control in patients with diabetes mellitus," *Am J Med Sci*. 343(2012):17–20.

Bolen, S., L. Feldman, J. Vassy, et al. "Systematic review: comparative effectiveness and safety of oral medications for type 2 diabetes mellitus," *Ann Intern Med*.147(2007):386–99.

Bosse, H. M., M. Nickel, S. Huwendiek, et al. "Peer role-play and standardised patients in communication training: A comparative study on the student perspective on acceptability, realism, and perceived effect," *BMC Med Educ* 10(2010):27.

Botelho, Richard J. "A negotiation model for the doctor-patient relationship," *Family Practice* 9 (1992) : 210–218. DOI: 10.1093/fampra/9.2.210.

Brawley, Otis W., "Prostate cancer screening: what we know, don't know, and believe," *Ann Intern Med*. 157(2012):135–36.

Brock, D. M., L. B. Mauksch, S. Witteborn, et al. "Effectiveness of intensive physician training in upfront agenda setting," *J Gen Intern Med*. 26(2011):1317–23.

Brown, Judith Belle, W. Wayne Weston, and Moira A. Stewart. "Patient-centred interviewing part II: Finding common ground," *Can Fam Physician* 35(1989): 153–157.

Calonge, N., D. B. Petitti, T. G. DeWitt, et al. "Screening for breast cancer: U.S. Preventive Services Task Force recommendation statement," *Annals of Internal Medicine* 151 (2009):716–26.

Campbell, Eric, Susan Regan, Russell Gruen, et al. "Professionalism in medicine: Results of a national survey of physicians," *Annals of Internal Medicine* 147 (2007):795–W234.

Caplan, Arthur. "Quantifying the efficacy of influenza vaccines," *Lancet Infectious Diseases* 12(2012):656–57.

Cassel Christine K. and James A. Guest. "Choosing wisely: Helping physicians and patients make smart decisions about their care," *Journal of the American Medical Association* 307(2012):1801–1802. DOI:10.1001/jama.2012.476.

Charon, Rita. "Narrative and medicine," *New England Journal of Medicine* 350(2004):862–4.

Chen, D.C. et al. "Characterizing changes in student empathy throughout medical school." *Medical Teaching* 34 (2012):305–11.

Chen, Pauline W. "Can Doctors Learn Empathy," *New York Times* Well blog, June 21, 2012, http://well.blogs.nytimes.com/2012/06/21/can-doctors-learn-empathy/. Accessed July 1, 2012.

Chisolm, Margaret S.and Constantine G. Lyketsos. *Systematic Psychiatric Evaluation.* Baltimore: Johns Hopkins University Press, 2012.

Cooper, L. A., D. Roter, and R. Johnson et al. "Patient-centered communication, ratings of care, and concordance of patient and physician race," *Annals of Internal Medicine* 139 (2003):907–15.

Cooper, L. A., D. L. Roter, K. A. Carson et al. "The associations of clinicians' implicit attitudes about race with medical visit communication and patient ratings of interpersonal care," *American Journal of Public Health* 102 (2012):979–87.

Cooper-Patrick, Lisa, Joseph J. Gallo, and Junius J. Gonzales. "Race, gender, and partnership in the physician-patient relationship," *JAMA*. 282(1999):583–89. doi:10.1001/jama.282.6.583.

Damasio, Antonio. *Descartes' Error: Emotion, Reason and the Human Brain.* New York: Random House, 2008.

DeBronkart, Dave. "Gimme My Damn Data," presentation at Medicine 2.0, 2009. Accessed http://www.slideshare.net/ePatientDave/gimme-my-damn-data-epatient-daves-keynote-at-medicine-20-2009 on December 3, 2012.

DeGroot, I. B., W. Otten, H. J. Smeets, et al. "Is the impact of hospital performance data greater in patients who have compared hospitals?," *BMC Health Services Research* 11(2011): 214.

Delbanco, Tom L. "Enriching the doctor-patient relationship by inviting the patient's perspective," *Ann Intern Med.* 116(1992):414–18.

Delbanco, Tom, Donald M. Berwick, and Jo Ivey Boufford. "Healthcare in a land called PeoplePower: nothing about me without me," *Health Expectations* 4(2001):144–50. DOI: 10.1046/j.1369-6513.2001.00145.x.

Detels, Roger , Alvaro Muñoz, Glen McFarlane, et al. For the Multicenter AIDS Cohort Study Investigators, "Effectiveness of potent antiretroviral therapy on time to AIDS and death in men with known HIV infection duration," *JAMA.* 280(1998):1497–1503. DOI:10-1001/pubs.JAMA-ISSN-0098-7484-280-17-joc72149.

Deveugele, Myriam, Anselm Derese, Atie van den Brink-Muinen, et al. "Consultation length in general practice: cross sectional study in six European countries," *BMJ* 325(2002). DOI: http://dx.doi.org/10.1136/bmj.325.7362.472.

Deveugele, M., et al. "Teaching communication skills to medical students, a challenge in the curriculum?" *Patient Education and Counseling* 58 (2005):265–70.

Diao, D., J. M. Wright, D. K. Cundiff, et al. "Pharmacotherapy for mild hypertension," *Cochrane Database Syst Rev* 8(2012):CD006742.

Dwan, K., D. G. Altman, J. A. Arnaiz, et al. "Systematic review of the empirical evidence of study publication bias and outcome reported bias," *PLoS ONE* 3(2008):e3081. DOI:10.1371/journal.pone.0003081.

Edelstein, Ludwig. "The Hippocratic oath: Text, translation, and interpretation," Baltimore: The Johns Hopkins University Press, 1964.

Epstein, Ronald M., Peter Franks, and Cleveland G. Shields "Patient-centered communication and diagnostic testing," *Ann Fam Med* 3(2005):415–421. DOI: 10.1370/afm.348.

Evans, H. M. "Wonder and the clinical encounter," Theor Med Bioeth (2012) 33:123–36, DOI 10.1007/s11017-012-9214-4.

Fayers, Peter M. and David Machin *"Quality of Life: The Assessment, Analysis, and Interpretation of Patient-Reported Outcomes"* New York: John Wiley & Sons, 2007.

Fisher, Elliot, David Wennberg, Therese Stukel, et al. "The implications of regional variations in Medicare spending, part 1: The content, quality, and accessibility of care, *Annals of Internal Medicine* 138(2003):273–87.

Fortess, Eric E. and Marshall B. Kapp, "Medical uncertainty, diagnostic testing, and legal liability," The *Journal of Law, Medicine & Ethics* 13(1985):213–18. DOI: 10.1111/j.1748-720X.1985.tb00925.x.

Fromme, E. K., D. Zive, T. A. Schmidt, et al. "POLST Registry do-not-resuscitate orders and other patient treatment preferences." *JAMA.* 307(2012):34–35.

Gawande, Atul. *The Checklist Manifesto: How to Get Things Right.* New York: Profile Books, 2010.

Gawande, Atul. *Complications.* New York: Metropolitan Books, 2002.

Glans, F., K. F. Eriksson, A. Segerström, et al., "Evaluation of the effects of exercise on insulin sensitivity in Arabian and Swedish women with type 2 diabetes," *Diabetes Res Clin Pract* 85(2009):69–74.

Good Stewardship Working Group, "The Top 5 Lists in Primary Care: meeting the responsibility of professionalism," *Archives of Internal Medicine* 171(2011):1385.

Gourlay, M. L., J. P. Fine, J. S. Preisser, et al. Study of Osteoporotic Fractures Research Group, "Bone-density testing interval and transition to osteoporosis in older women," *New England Journal of Medicine* 366 (2012):225–33.

Grayson, Martha S., Dale A. Newton, and Lori F. Thompson, "Payback time: The associations of debt and income with medical student career choice," *Medical Education* 46(2012):983–91. DOI: 10.1111/j.1365-2923.2012.04340.x.

Groopman, Jerome. *How Doctors Think.* New York: Houghton Mifflin Harcourt, 2007.

Groopman Jerome and Pamela Hartzband, *Your Medical Mind: How to Decide What is Right for You.* New York: Penguin Press, 2011.

Haley, N., B. Maheux, M. Rivard, et al. "Sexual health risk assessment and counseling in primary care: How involved are general practitioners and obstetrician-gynecologists?" *Am J Public Health.* 89(1999):899–902.

Hanyok L.A. et al. "Practicing patient-centered care: The questions clinically excellent physicians use to get to know their patients as individuals," *The Patient* 5 (2012):141–45.

Harris, Gardner. "New for aspiring doctors, the people skills test," *New York Times*, July 10, 2011.

Hofmann, J. C., N. S. Wenger, R. B. Davis, et al. "Patient preferences for communication with physicians about end-of-life decisions," *Annals of Internal Medicine* 127 (1997):1–12.

Hsu, I. et al. "Providing support to patients in emotional encounters: A new perspective on missed empathic opportunities," *Patient Education and Counseling* 2012 Jul 17.

Hughes, J. "Organization and Information at the Bed-Side: The Experience of the Medical Division of Labor by University Hospitals' Inpatients" (PhD diss., University of Chicago, 1994). http://www.changesurfer.com/Hlth/HuDiss.html. Accessed June 19, 2012.

Hughes, S., D. Cohen, "A systematic review of long-term studies of drug treated and non-drug treated depression," *J Affect Disord.* 118(2009):9–18.

Huynh, Phuong Trang, Cathy Schoen, Robin Osborn, et al., "The U.S. health care divide: Disparities in primary care experiences by income," (2006) The Commonwealth Fund. http://www.commonwealthfund.org/Publications/Fund-Reports/2006/Apr/The-U-S-Health-Care-Divide-Disparities-in-Primary-Care-Experiences-by-Income.aspx. Accessed December 4, 2012.

Inzucchi, S. E., R. M. Bergenstal, J. B. Buse, et al. "Management of hyperglycemia in type 2 diabetes: A patient centered approach. Position Statement of the American Diabetes Association (ADA) and the European Association for the Study of Diabetes (EASD)," *Diabetes Care* 35 (2012):1364-79.

Israel Barbara A., et al. "Review of community-based research: Assessing partnership–based approaches to improve public health," *Annual Review of Public Health* 19 (1998):173–202.

Jackson, J. L., K. Kroenke. "The effect of unmet expectations among adults presenting with physical symptoms," *Ann Intern Med* 134(2001):889–97.

Jacobs, W. C., M. P. Arts, M. W. van Tulder, et al. "Surgical techniques for sciatica due to herniated disc, a systematic review," Eur Spine J. July 20, 2012.

Jerant, A., P. Franks, R. L. Kravitz "Associations between pain control self-efficacy, self-efficacy for communicating with physicians, and subsequent pain severity among cancer patients," *Patient Educ Couns.* 85(2011):275–80.

Joffe, S., M. Manocchia, J. C. Weeks, et al., "What do patients value in their hospital care? An empirical perspective on autonomy centred bioethics," *J Med Ethics* 29(2003):103–8.

Joynt, K. E., E. J. Orav, A. K. Jha. "The association between hospital volume and processes, outcomes, and costs of care for congestive heart failure," *Ann Intern Med* 154(2011): 94–102, DOI: 10.1059/0003-4819-154-2-201101180-00008.

Kaba, R. and P. Sooniakumaran, "The evolution of the doctor-patient relationship," *International Journal of Surgery* 5 (2007): 57. http://dx.doi.org/10.1016/j.ijsu.2006.01.005.

Kagawa-Singer, Marjorie and Shaheen Kassim-Lakha, "A Strategy to Reduce Cross-cultural Miscommunication and Increase the Likelihood of Improving Health Outcomes," *Academic Medicine* 78 (2003):577–87.

Kahneman, Daniel. "A different approach to health state valuation," *Value in Health* 12(2009):516–17.

Kandula, Namratha R., Neerja R. Khurana, Gregory Makoul, et al. "A community and culture-centered approach to developing effective cardiovascular health messages," *Journal of General Internal Medicine* 27(2012):1308–16.

Kravitz, R. L., R. A. Bell, C. E. Franz, " A taxonomy of requests by patients (TORP): A new system for understanding clinical negotiation in office practice," *Journal of Family Practice* 48(1999):872–78.

Laakso, M., H. Cederberg, "Glucose control in diabetes: Which target level to aim for?" *Journal of Internal Medicine* 272(2012):1–12. DOI: 10.1111/j.1365-2796.2012.02528.x.

Laine, Christine. "The annual physical examination: needless ritual or necessary routine?" *Annals of Internal Medicine* 136(2002):701–3.

Lenzer, Jeanne. "Cochrane review finds no proved benefit in drug treatment for patients with mild hypertension," *BMJ* 2012:345. DOI: http://dx.doi.org/10.1136/bmj.e5511.

Levinson, W., A. Kao, A. Kuby, et al. "Not all patients want to participate in decision making. A national study of public preferences," *J Gen Intern Med* 20(2005):531–35. DOI: 10.1111/j.1525-1497.2005.04101.x.

Lipkin Jr. M., S. M. Putnam, and J. Lazare, editors. *The Medical Interview*. New York: Springer, 1994.

Luft, Harold S., Deborah W. Garnick, David H. Mark, et al. "Does Quality Influence Choice of Hospital?" *Journal of the American Medical Association* 263(1990):2899–2906. DOI:10.1001/jama.1990.03440210049031.

Lynn, Joanne, Janice Lynch Schuster, and Joan Harrold. *Handbook for Mortals: Guidance for People Facing Serious Illness*. New York: Oxford University Press, 2011.

Makary, Martin. *Unaccountable: What Hospitals Won't Tell You and How Transparency Can Revolutionize Health Care*. New York: Bloomsbury Press, 2012.

Marvel, M. K., R. M. Epstein, K. Flowers, et al. "Soliciting the patient's agenda: Have we improved?," *JAMA* 281(1999):283–87.

McNamara, Judith R., G. Russell Warnick, and Gerald R. Cooper. "A brief history of lipid and lipoprotein measurements and their contribution to clinical chemistry," *Clinica Chimica Acta* 369(2006):158–67.

"Medicare Program; Revisions to Payment Policies Under the Physician Fee Schedule, DME Face-to-Face Encounters, Elimination of the Requirement for Termination of Non-Random Prepayment Complex Medical Review and Other Revisions to Part B for CY 2013," *Federal Register* 77(2012): 68891–69373. http://www.gpo.gov/fdsys/pkg/FR-2012-11-16/pdf/2012-26900.pdf. Accessed December 4, 2012.

Miller, William R., Steven P. Rollnick. *Motivational Interviewing, Preparing People for Change*. New York: Guilford Press, 2002.

Misch, Donald A. "Evaluating physicians' professionalism and humanism: The case for humanism 'connoisseurs,'" *Academic Medicine* 77 (2002):489–95.

Montgomery, A. A., J. Harding, and T. Fahey. "Shared decision making in hypertension: The impact of patient preferences on treatment choice," *Family Practice* 18 (2001):309–13.

Morgan, Myfanwy and C. J. Watkins "Managing hypertension: beliefs and responses to medication among cultural groups," *Sociology of Health & Illness* 10(1998):561–78.

Morrell, D. C., M. E. Evans, R. W. Morris, et al. "The "five minute" consultation: effect of time constraint on clinical content and patient satisfaction," *Br Med J* (Clin Res Ed) 292(1986). DOI: http://dx.doi.org/10.1136/bmj.292.6524.870.

Morrison, W. "Is that all you got?" *J Palliat Med* 13(2010):1384–85.

Morsi, E., P. K. Lindenauer, and M. B. Rothberg. "Primary care physicians' use of publicly reported quality data in hospital referral decisions," *Journal of Hospital Medicine* 7(2012): 370–75, DOI: 10.1002/jhm.1931.

Moyer, Virginia A. "Screening for prostate cancer: U.S. Preventive Services Task Force recommendation statement," *Annals of Internal Medicine* 157(2012):120–34.

Nabel Elizabeth G. and Eugene Braunwald. "A tale of coronary artery disease and myocardial infarction," *N Engl J Med* 366(2012):54–63. DOI: 10.1056/NEJMra1112570.

Nelson, H. D., K. Tyne, and A. Naik "Screening for breast cancer: Systematic evidence review update for the US Preventive Services Task Force," *Ann Intern Med.* 151(2009): 727–W242. DOI: 10.1059/0003-4819-151-10-200911170-00009.

Nuland, Sherwin. *How We Die: Reflections on Life's Final Chapter*. New York: Random House, 2000.

Ockene, Judith K., Jean Kristeller, Robert Goldberg, et al. "Increasing the efficacy of physician-delivered smoking interventions," *Journal of General Internal Medicine* 6(1991):1–8.

Osterholme, Michael, Nicholas Kelley, Alfred Sommer, et al., "Efficacy and effectiveness of influenza vaccines: a systematic review and meta-analysis," *Lancet Infectious Diseases* 12(2011):36–44.

Pope, G. C., J. E. Schneider, "Trends in physician income," *Health Affairs* 11(1992):181–93. DOI: 10.1377/hlthaff.11.1.181.

Pronovost, Peter and Eric Vohr, *Safe Patients, Smart Hospitals: How One Doctor's Checklist Can Help Change Healthcare From the Inside Out.* New York: Penguin, 2010.

Qaseem, Amir, Patrick Alguire, Paul Dallas, et al. "Appropriate use of screening and diagnostic tests to foster high-value, cost-conscious care," *Ann Intern Med.*156(2012):147–49.

Ray, Gretchen M., James J. Nawarskas, and Joe R. Anderson. "Blood pressure monitoring technique impacts hypertension treatment," *Journal of General Internal Medicine* 27(2012):623–29. DOI: 10.1007/s11606-011-1937-9.

Read, S., M. King, J. Watson. "Sexual dysfunction in primary medical care: prevalence, characteristics and detection by the general practitioner," *J Public Health Med.* 19(1997):387–91.

Reuben David B. and Mary E. Tinetti, "Goal-Oriented patient care—an alternative health outcomes paradigm," *New England Journal of Medicine* 366 (2012):777–79.

Rider, E. A., M. M. Hinrichs, and B. A. Lown, "A model for communication skills assessment across the undergraduate curriculum," *Med Teach* 28(2006):127–34.

Rittenhouse, Diane R. "The patient centered medical home: Will it stand the test of health reform?" *JAMA* 301 (2009):2038–40.

Rogers, Carl R. "The necessary and sufficient conditions of therapeutic personality change," *Journal of Consulting Psychiatry* 21(1957):95–103.

Rosseau, Paul. "Empathy," *Journal of Hospital and Palliative Care* 25 (2008):261–62, DOI: 10.1177/1049909108315524AM.

Roter, D. L. and J. A. Hall. "Physician gender and patient-centered communication: A critical review of empirical research," *Annu Rev Public Health* 25(2004):497–519.

Roter, D. L., M. Stewart, S. M. Putnam, M. Lipkin Jr., W. Stiles, andT. S. Inui. "Communication patterns of primary care physicians," *JAMA* 277 (1997):350–56.

Roter, Debra and Judith A. Hall. *Doctors Talking to Patients/Patients Talking to Doctors.* Westport, CT: Greenwood Publishing Group, 2006.

Rubak, S., A. Sandbaek, T. Lauritzen, and B. Christensen. "Motivational interviewing: A systematic review and meta-analysis," *Br J Gen Pract.* 55(2005):305–12.

Ruggiero, Laurie, Amparo Castillo, Lauretta Quinn and Michelle Hochwert. "Translation of the Diabetes Prevention Program's Lifestyle Intervention: Role of Community Health Workers," *Current Diabetes Reports* 2012, 12:127–37. DOI: 10.1007/s11892-012-0254-y.

Rusk, Howard and Jason Novey. "The effect of chronic illness on families," *Marriage and Family Living* 1957;193–97.

Ryan, Mandy and Shelley Farrar, "Using conjoint analysis to elicit preferences for health care," *British Medical Journal* 320(2000):1530–33.

Sasson, Comilla, David J. Magid, Paul Chan, et al. "Association of neighborhood characteristics with bystander-initiated CPR," *N Engl J Med* 367(2012):1607–15.

Schneider, Carl. *The Practice of Autonomy: Patients, Doctors, and Medical Decisions."* New York: Oxford University Press, 1998.

Schoen, Cathy, Robin Osborn, Michelle M. Doty, et al. "Toward higher-performance health systems: Adults' health care experiences in seven countries, 2007," *Health Aff* 26(2007):w717–w734, DOI: 10.1377/hlthaff.26.6.w717.

Seabury, Seth A., Anupam B. Jena, and Amitabh Chandra. "Trends in the earnings of health care professionals in the United States, 1987–2010," *JAMA.* 308(2012):2083–85. DOI:10.1001/jama.2012.14552.

Sehgal, Ashwini. "The role of reputation in *U.S News & World Report*'s rankings of the top 50 American hospitals," *Annals of Internal Medicine* 152(2010):521–25.

Singer, P. A., E. S. Tasch, C. Stocking, et al. "Sex or survival: Trade-offs between quality and quantity of life. *J Clin Oncol* 9(1991):328–34.

Skloot, Rebecca. *The Immortal Life of Henrietta Lacks.* New York: Macmillan, 2010.

Smith, Robert A., Vilma Cokkinides, Durado Brooks, et al. "Cancer screening in the United States, 2010: A review of current American Cancer Society guidelines and issues in cancer screening," *CA* 60(2010). DOI: 10.3322/caac.20063.

Sparrenberger, F., F. T., Cichelero, A. M. Fonseca, et al. "Does psychosocial stress cause hypertension? A systematic review of observational studies," *J Hum Hypertens.* 23(2009):12–9.

Srinivas, S. V., R. A. Deyo, Z. D. Berger, "Application of "less is more" to low back pain," *Arch Intern Med* 172(2012):1016–20.

Stafford, R. S. "Off-Label use of drugs and medical devices: A review of policy implications," *Clinical Pharmacology & Therapeutics* (2012); advance online publication 4 April 2012. DOI:10.1038/clpt.2012.22.

Stevanovic, Gordana, Gordana Tucakovic, Rajko Dotlic, and Vladimir Kanjuh, "Correlation of clinical diagnoses with autopsy findings: A retrospective study of 2,145 consecutive autopsies," *Human Pathology* 17(1986):1225–30.

Strull, W. M., B. Lo, G. Charles, "Do patients want to participate in medical decision making?" *Journal of the American Medical Association* 252 (1984):2990–94.

Suchman, A. L. and D. A. Matthews. "What makes the patient-doctor relationship therapeutic? Exploring the connexional dimension of medical care," *Ann Intern Med* 108 (1988):125.

Sulmasy, D. P., L. Snyder "Substituted interests and best judgments: an integrated model of surrogate decision making," *JAMA* 304(2010):1946–47.

Szasz, Thomas S. and Marc H. Hollender. "The basic models of the doctor-patient relationship," *Archives of Internal Medicine* 97 (1956):585.

Szasz, Thomas S., William F. Knoff and Marc H. Hollender, "The doctor-patient relationship and its historical context," Am J Psychiatry 115 (1958):522–28.

Thombs, Brett D., James C. Coyne, Pim Cuijpers, et al. "Rethinking recommendations for screening for depression in primary care," *CMAJ* 184(2012):413–18.

Thorpe, C. T., L. E. Fahey, H. Johnson, "Facilitating healthy coping in patients with diabetes: A systematic review," Diabetes Educ Oct 16, 2012. DOI: 10.1177/0145721712464400.

Trivedi, Madhukar H., A. John Rush, Stephen R. Wisniewski, et al. For the STAR*D Study Team, "Evaluation of outcomes with citalopram for depression using measurement-based care in STAR*D: Implications for clinical practice," Am J Psychiatry 163(2006):28–40. 10.1176/appi.ajp.163.1.28.Urban, Linei and Cicero Urban." Role of mammography versus magnetic resonance imaging for breast cancer screening," *Current Breast Cancer Reports* 2012, http://dx.doi.org/10.1007/s12609-012-0085-5.

Vastine, A., J. Gittelsohn, B. Ethelbah, et al. "Formative research and stakeholder participation in intervention development," *Am J Health Behav* 29(2005):57–69.

Vig, E. K., H. Starks, J. S. Taylor, et al. "Surviving surrogate decision-making: What helps and hampers the experience of making medical decisions for others," *J Gen Intern Med.* 22(2007):1274–79.

Wagner, P., J. Hendrich, G. Moseley, and V. Hudson, "Defining medical professionalism: a qualitative study," *Medical Education* 41 (2007):288–94.

Walker, Jan, Immy Holloway, and Beatrice Sofaer, "In the system: the lived experience of chronic back pain from the perspectives of those seeking help from pain clinics," *Pain* 80(1999):621–28, http://dx.doi.org/10.1016/S0304-3959(98)00254-1.

Walsh, James J. "Psychotherapy: What the modern physician thinks of the mind cure as practised in all ages," *The Independent*, September 11, 1913, p.628, http://books.google.com/books/download/The_Independent.pdf?id=6Pi0AAAAMAAJ&output=pdf&sig=ACfU3U2E0VFgf0f0o79itkYoWTho329JYg.

Walter, F.M., J. Emery. "Perceptions of family history across common diseases: a qualitative study in primary care," *Fam Pract.* 23(2006):472–80.

Warwick, H. M. and P. M. Salkovskis. "Reassurance," *British Medical Journal* (Clinical Research Edition), 290(1985): 1028.

Weeks, Jane C., Paul J. Catalano, Angel Cronin, et al. "Patients' expectations about effects of chemotherapy for advanced cancer," *N Engl J Med* 367(2012):1616–25. DOI: 10.1056/NEJMoa1204410.

Whitehead, W. E. "Diagnosing and managing fecal incontinence: If you don't ask, they won't tell," *Gastroenterology* 129(2005):6.

Wilt, Timothy J., Michael K. Brawer, Karen M. Jones, et al. For the PIVOT Study Group. "Radical prostatectomy versus observation for localized prostate cancer," *New England Journal of Medicine* 367(2012):203–13. DOI: 10.1056/NEJMoa1113162.

Wolff, S. H. and R. Harris, "The harms of testing: new attention to an old concern," *Journal of the American Medical Association*, 307(2012):565–66.

Woloshin, Steven and Lisa M. Schwartz. "How a charity oversells mammography," *British Medical Journal* 2012;345.

Wooten, Karen G., Pascale M. Wortley, James A. Singleton, et al. "Perceptions matter: Beliefs about influenza vaccine and vaccination behavior among elderly white, black and Hispanic Americans," *Vaccine* 30(2012):6927–34.

Wray, R. J., K. Jupka, W. Ross, et al. "How can you improve vaccination rates among older AfricanAmericans?," *J Fam Pract*, 56 (2007):925–29.

Yin, M., S. Bastacky, U. Chandran, M. J. Becich and R. Dhir. "Prevalence of incidentalprostate cancer in the general population: A study of healthy organ donors," *Journal Urology* 179 (2008):892–95.

Yuen, J. K., M. C. Reid, M. D. Fetters. "Hospital do-not-resuscitate orders: Why they have failed and how to fix them," *Journal Gen Intern Med.* 26(2011):791–97.

Index

Accountable Carganizations (ACOs), 76, 173
adverse effects, 156–158
Affordable Care Act, 7, 76, 172; Independent Payment Advisory Board and, 155
African Americans, 23
agendas, xiii, 78, 104; addressing explicitly, 107, 107; negotiating, 107; and testing, 160–162; and time, 106
agenda-setting. *See* agendas
American Academy of Family Practice, 171
anxiety disorder, 135
autonomy, 175n3, 190

back pain, 110; imaging studies in, 110–111, 152–153, 160, 166
Balint, Michael, 25
Balint groups, 25–26
Baltimore, xi, 21, 23
barriers between patient and doctor, 88; role of culture in overcoming, 91
Beach, Mary Catherine, 77
behavior change, 118
Bellevue Hospital, 1, 3, 21
Best Hospitals in America. See U.S. News
bias. *See also* racial bias: cognitive bias, 114
Bishop, Scott, 17
blood tests, 160; for cholesterol, 160

bone mineral scans, 37, 165
body language. *See* non-verbal communication
Botelho, Richard, 107
bowel complaints, 129
breast cancer, screening for. *See* mammography

Campbell, Eric, 38
cancer: cervical cancer, 153; metastatic, 153; prostate cancer, 30–31
Caplan, Arthur, 141
cardiopulmonary resuscitation (CPR): neighborhoods and, 143
care coordination, 168
checklists, 52
chemotherapy, 53
choreography, 19
circumcision: metzitzah b'peh, sucking the wound in, 146
cognitive science: and diagnostic reasoning, 115
common ground: and culture, 95; and end-of-life decision making, 97; and everyday conversations, 98
communication: before the visit, 63; patient-doctor communication, 22
communities: health of, xiii, 140; empowerment of, 144–146, 149
compliance: lack of, 18
Consumer Reports, 55

Cooper, Lisa, 16
cultural competency, 16
culture, 91, 92; in the doctor's office, 93; universal aspects of, 92

data: "Gimme my damn data!", 87, 163; open access to, 87–88
death. *See also* end of life: talking about, 131
decision making, 124
depression, 123–124, 135, 154
diabetes, 46–47, 53, 54, 59, 103, 109, 154; community health in, 148; diet and, 49; hemoglobin A1C targets and, 169–170
disparities, 8
diversity: of people, 1; of languages, 1
doctor appointment, 68
doctor salaries. *See* financial incentives
doctor visit. *See* doctor-patient interview
doctor-patient communication, 59, 76, 176n7; and chronic illness, 176n9; in the hospital, 89–90; non-verbal, 84; science of, xii, 89; sensitive issues and, 137–138
doctor-patient interview: agenda-setting in, 30; as procedure, 2; cues in, 80; different priorities in, reconciling, 103; flow in, 17; goals of, 101; history in, 28; interval between, 72; introduction in, 29; length of, 11–12; long-term health goals and, 74; mindfulness in, 81; opening question in, 19; parts of, 28, 28–29; physical exam in, 28; plan afterwards, 70, 71; problem solving in, 81; questions in, 32; race in, 16, 29; three functions of, 5, 13; time for, xii, 71
doctor-patient relationship, 24, 25; doctors' needs in, 47; roles in, 27, 48; screening tests and, 167; types of, 27

Edelstein, Ludwig, 50
electrocardiograms, 160
electronic medical record, 69
emotion, 80; anger, 119; and cognition, 114; fear, 121; in the doctor-patient interview, 113; in medical education, 80; sadness, 123

empathy, 49, 78, 79; artificial or feigned empathy, 78
empowerment, 6
end-of-life care, 92–93, 97; decisions and, 131; and the doctor-patient relationship, 133; protocols and, 131; Physician Orders for Life Sustaining Treatment (POLST) and, 131; surrogates and, 135; values and, 131–132
explanatory models, 140, 141

financial incentives, 8, 9, 171
framing, 64, 65

Gawande, Atul, 52
Groopman, Jerome, 114, 151
guidelines, 109

Hall, Judith A., 11
Hartzband, Pamela, 151
HCAHPS (Hospital Care Quality Information from the Consumer Perspective), 58
health beliefs. *See* explanatory models
health care system, xi; payment structure of, 172; reform of, xiii, 7–2, 155
health problems: expressing them, 63
heart disease, 153; risk of, 59
HEDIS (Healthcare Effectiveness Data and Information Set), 61
high blood pressure, 3, 13–14, 15, 35, 61, 93, 98–99; community-based interventions and, 94; measuring technique, 61; and stress, 93
history of medicine, 23
history taking. *See* doctor-patient interview
HIV/AIDS, 77, 104, 153
Hippocratic Oath, 37–38, 50
Hollender, Marc, 27
honesty, 36
Hospital Compare (Center for Medicare and Medicaid Services), 55
hospitalization: reason for, 89–90
Hughes, James J., 26
hypertension. *See* high blood pressure

Implicit Association Test. *See* racial bias
incentives: for developing a relationship between patient and doctor, 173

incontinence: fecal, 129; urinary, 129
inequities in health care, 16
insurance companies, 8
integrity and meaning, 95
interview. *See* doctor-patient interview

Johns Hopkins Hospital, xi, 7, 21, 55

Kagawa-Singer, Marjorie, 91
Kassim-Lakha, Shaeen, 91
Knoff, William F., 27
Kravitz, R. J., 108

laboratory tests, 84, 167
language: language of the doctor and
    language of the patient, differences in,
    109
languages, 1
Lau, Mark, 17
Lipkin, Mack Jr., MD, 2, 5, 13
Luft, Howard, 57
Lynne, Joanne, 19

mammography, 37, 53, 166
medical education, 75; biomedical model
    in, 75, 79, 114
medication, 84; experiences with, 69–70;
    not taking medication as prescribed, 18,
    84; records of, 69; refills of, 84
mental health, 135
mindfulness, xii, 13, 17, 81
motivational interviewing, 116; smoking
    cessation counseling using, 116

National Physicians Alliance, 160
negotiation, 15
New York City, xi, 1; Department of
    Health and Mental Hygiene, 146
New York University, 89
non-verbal communication, 84
"nothing about me, without me", 163

Obamacare. *See* Affordable Care Act
open-endedness, 13
Osler, Sir William, 22
overuse, 149, 152, 155; screening tests and,
    160, 166; variation in care in, 159

pain. *See also* back pain: chronic pain, 53

paperwork, 69
Parsons, Talcott, 26
paternalism, 6
The Patient Interview, 5
patient-centered decision making, 31, 32
patient-centered medical home, 76
Patient-Centered Outcomes Research
    Institute, 7
patient-centered care, 6, 8, 22–23
Patient Protection and Affordable Care Act
    of 2010. *See* Affordable Care Act
patient-reported outcomes. *See* Quality
patient safety. *See* Quality
patients: as self-advocates, 83; difficult, 5
physical exam. *See* doctor-patient
    interview
Physician Orders for Life Sustaining
    Treatment (POLST), 131
post-partum, 4
The Practice of Autonomy, 6
preferences, 31
primary care, 1, 3, 8–9, 21
primary care providers, payment of, 171
professionalism, 37–50
Pronovost, Peter, 52, 59
prostate cancer, 36, 149, 151, 177n3
public health, 9, 139

quality, 51, 60; of hospitals, 56–57,
    178n11; of life, measurement of, 155;
    measuring, flaws of, 57; process
    measures of, 51–52; process versus
    outcome in measuring, 52–53, 55;
    patient-reported outcomes in, 54, 55;
    patient safety in, 55; regulations and,
    60, 147
questions: asking, in medical visit, 32;
    general opening, 104; open-ended and
    closed-ended, 78; starter questions, list
    of, 99

racial bias: of doctors, 29, 49, 144, 188
randomized controlled trials, 5
rationing, 173
regard: unconditional positive regard,
    doctors for patients, 115
regulations, 60
relationship: doctor-patient relationship
    and mental health, 135

reputation, 56
requests: by patients, taxonomy of, 108; requests for information and requests for action, 108
roles: of doctor, 78; of patient and doctor, 45
Roter, Debra, 11, 77
Roter Interaction Analysis System (RIAS), 77
RUC (Specialty Society Relative Value Scale Update Committee), 8, 171

Schneider, Carl, 6
Sehgal, Ashwini, 56
self-advocacy, xi
sex, 130; personal history of, in the visit, 130; specific problems with, 130
shared decision making, 154; barriers to, 164–165; patients' preferences regarding, 163
Smith, Stephen, 160
smoking cessation, 3, 175n1
social media, 163
Southeast Asians, 140–141
Specialty Society Relative Value Scale Update Committee. *See* RUC
Strull, William, 32
Suchman, Andrew, 79

Sulmasy, Daniel, 131
symptom diary. *See* symptoms
symptoms. *See also* individual symptoms: diary of, 66, 137; narrative in, 67; presentation of,. *See* See also framing 66; recording, 66
Szasz, Thomas, 27

telephone: making a doctor appointment by, 68
time: clock time versus visit time, 12
Tisch Hospital, 2
Top 5 project, 160

Ultra Orthodox Jews, 147
uncertainty, 35–36
uncomfortable topics, 128
United States Preventive Services Task Force (USPSTF), recommendations of, 151
urine tests, 160
U.S. News, 55

vaccinations, 140, 141–142; influenza vaccine, 141

wonder, 15